Evidence-based Resource in Anaesthesia and Analgesia

Second edition

Evidence-based Resource in Anaesthesia and Analgesia

Second edition

Edited by

Martin R Tramèr

Division of Anaesthesiology, Geneva University Hospitals,
University of Geneva, Geneva, Switzerland

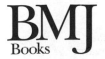

First published in 2000
Second impression 2002
Second edition 2003
by BMJ Books, BMA House, Tavistock Square,
London WC1H 9JR

www.bmjbooks.com
www.evidbasedanaesth.com

British Library Cataloguing in Publication Data

A catalogue record for this book is available from the British Library

ISBN 0 7279 1786 2

Typeset by SIVA Math Setters, Chennai, India
Printed and bound in Spain by GraphyCems, Navarra

Contents

Part III: Dissemination, implementation, and research agenda

Contributors

Peter T-L Choi
Assistant Professor, Departments of Anesthesia and Clinical Epidemiology and Biostatistics, McMaster University, Hamilton, Ontario, Canada

Mehrengise K Cooper
Fellow in Paediatric Intensive Care, Paediatric Intensive Care Unit Office, The Hospital for Sick Children, Great Ormond Street, London, UK

Jørgen B Dahl
Chairman, Department of Anaesthesia, Glostrup University Hospital, Glostrup, Denmark

Tony Gin
Professor and Chairman, Department of Anaesthesia and Intensive Care, The Chinese University of Hong Kong, Prince of Wales Hospital, Shatin, NT, Hong Kong, China

Neville W Goodman
Consultant Anaesthetist, Department of Anaesthesia, Southmead Hospital, Bristol, UK

Kathrine Holte
Research Fellow, Department of Surgical Gastroenterology, Hvidovre University Hospital, Hvidovre, Denmark

Stephen Halpern
Departments of Anaesthesiology and Obstetrics and Gynaecology, University of Toronto, Ontario, Canada

Henrik Kehlet
Professor of Surgery, Department of Surgical Gastroenterology, Hvidovre University Hospital, Hvidovre, Denmark

Anna Lee
Assistant Professor, Department of Anaesthesia and Intensive Care, The Chinese University of Hong Kong, Prince of Wales Hospital, Shatin, NT, Hong Kong, China

Barbara Leighton
Professor of Anesthesiology, Professor of Obstetrics and Gynecology, Chief, Section of Obstetric Anesthesiology, Washington University School of Medicine, St Louis, Missouri, USA

Henry J McQuay
Professor for Pain Relief, Pain Research, Nuffield Department of Anaesthetics, University of Oxford, The Churchill, Oxford Radcliffe Hospital, Headington, Oxford, UK

Steen Møiniche
Staff Anaesthetist, Department of Anaesthesia, Glostrup University Hospital, Glostrup, Denmark

R Andrew Moore
Editor Bandolier, Pain Research, Nuffield Department of Anaesthetics, University of Oxford, Radcliffe Oxford Hospitals, The Churchill, Oxford, UK

Paul S Myles
Head of Research and Associate Professor, Department of Anaesthesia and Pain Management, Alfred Hospital, Melbourne, Departments of Anaesthesia, and Epidemiology and Preventive Medicine, Monash University, Melbourne and National Health and Medical Research Practitioner Fellow, Canberra, Australia

Tom Pedersen
Chairman, Department of Anaesthesiology, and Co-ordinating Editor of the Cochrane Anaesthesia Review Group, Bispebjerg University Hospital, Copenhagen, Denmark

Ceri J Phillips
Reader in Health Economics, Centre for Health Economics and Policy Studies, School of Health Science, University of Wales Swansea, Singleton Park, Swansea, UK

Adrienne G Randolph
Multidisciplinary Intensive Care Unit, Department of Anesthesia, Children's Hospital, Boston and Harvard Medical School, Boston, Massachusetts, USA

Martin R Tramèr
Staff Anaesthetist, Division of Anaesthesiology, Department of Anaesthesiology, Pharmacology and Surgical Intensive Care, Geneva University Hospitals, Privat-Docent at the Faculty of Medicine, University of Geneva, Geneva, Switzerland

Bernhard Walder
Staff Anaesthetist, Division of Anaesthesiology, Department of Anaesthesiology, Pharmacology and Surgical Intensive Care, Geneva University Hospitals, Privat-Docent at the Faculty of Medicine, University of Geneva, Geneva, Switzerland

Introduction

This is the second edition of the first book on evidence-based anaesthesia and analgesia. Those who have read the first edition[1] know that this is not a conventional textbook. And those who are looking for authoritative opinion, eminence-based doctrine, and cookbook medicine will definitely be disappointed. This book is about best-evidence data in anaesthesia, pain treatment, and critical care, about dissemination of these data, and about implementation of data into daily clinical practice. We tried hard to provide both methodological and clinical messages, and to formulate valid guidelines whenever feasible.

This second edition is both an update and a further development of the first. Obviously, the volume of the book has increased, as many more high-quality systematic reviews that critically appraise and summarise the relevant and valid literature have been published in the past few years. Authors from Australia, Canada, Denmark, Hong Kong, the United Kingdom, the United States, and Switzerland have participated in writing this book. Little attempt was made to standardise the composition and the style of the chapters, and so each chapter reflects the author's personal style.

The book has been divided into three parts. The first part starts with Nev Goodman's critical appraisal of evidence-based medicine. Then, Paul Myles presents the strengths of large randomised trials, and Andrew Moore does the same for systematic reviews and meta-analyses.

The second part of the book is on clinical application of best-evidence data. The topics fitted the criteria for inclusion if they were related to anaesthesia, pain treatment, or critical care, and had been discussed in several published systematic reviews. This does not mean that other subjects are less important; it only indicates either that other subjects have not (yet) been studied with the same systematic scientific rigour, or that we were unable to find an author to write a relevant chapter. In the first edition, there were five clinically oriented chapters, and three of those were on postoperative pain treatment. Now, the reader will find seven chapters in that part of the book, only two of which are on postoperative pain treatment. We had long discussions about whether or not we should change the title of the book to *Evidence-based Resource in Perioperative Medicine*. We eventually decided to stay with the original title, knowing that in many countries perioperative medicine is a subheading of anaesthesia, rather than *vice versa*.

The chapters on central venous catheters (by Mehrengise Cooper and Adrienne Randolph), intravenous fluids for resuscitation (by Peter Choi), and propofol for sedation and anaesthesia (by Bernhard Walder and Martin Tramèr) indicate that the book has widened its spectrum to include evidence-based critical care. Chapters relevant to postoperative pain treatment include an overview on the usefulness of peripheral analgesia (by Steen Møiniche and Jørgen Dahl) and Henry McQuay's update on acute pain, with special reference to oral analgesics. Stephen Halpern and Barbara Leighton wrote the chapter on the role of epidurals for labour. Finally, Martin Tramèr updated the chapter on prevention and treatment of postoperative nausea and vomiting. Unfortunately, we were unable to motivate anybody to write an update on transfusions; interested readers are referred to the first edition of the book.[1]

The third part of the book is about dissemination, implementation, health economy, and research agenda. Dissemination and implementation of scientific data are becoming increasingly important. Great advances have been made in designing and conducting valid clinical trials and in performing powerful systematic reviews. Evidence-based medicine, however, is not only about creating new valid scientific knowledge or about systematically searching and appraising existing contemporaneous research findings; it is also about using these data as the basis for making clinical decisions.[2] There is a need for innovation to make high-quality data comprehensible, to transfer the data to the clinician, and to motivate clinicians to accept a change in daily clinical practice towards improved and safer patient care. The Cochrane Collaboration plays a role in this process; Tom Pedersen, in his chapter, presents the Cochrane Anaesthesia Review Group.[3] Anna Lee and Tony Gin present models to facilitate the application of the aggregate results of quantitative systematic reviews to the individual patient level.

Economic constraints are increasingly interacting with clinicians' freedom to use their favourite interventions. However, what we like most is not necessarily the best for our patients. For each intervention – prophylactic, therapeutic, or diagnostic – the gold standard – the most efficacious, the least harmful, and the cheapest – needs to be identified.[4] Ceri Phillips' chapter is an easily understandable introduction into health economics and cost effectiveness.

Last, but not least, systematic reviews are important tools for defining rational, and thus ethical, research agendas. They tell us what we know and, as a consequence, what we don't know. Thus, research protocols that are submitted to ethical committees should ideally be accompanied by a systematic review of the relevant literature, to strengthen the rationale behind the planned scientific project and to justify the design of the study. The chapter by Kathrine

Holte and Henrik Kehlet is a powerful example of this; on the basis of data from large randomised trials and from systematic reviews, the authors explain how future clinical research in the field of epidural analgesia should be designed, and what should be avoided.

We abstained from again including a comprehensive list of systematic reviews that are relevant to healthcare providers in anaesthesia, pain treatment, and critical care. In the first edition of the book, that list contained almost 100 titles.[1] Today, more than 300 relevant references can be accessed through the web page of the Geneva Evidence-based Perioperative Medicine Group;[5] the group takes due care to update the list periodically.

Martin R Tramèr

References

1. Tramèr MR, ed. *Evidence based resource in anaesthesia and analgesia.* London: BMJ Publishing Group, 2000.
2. Rosenberg W, Donald A. Evidence based medicine: an approach to clinical problem solving. *BMJ* 1995;**310**:1122–6.
3. The Cochrane Anaesthesia Review Group. http://www.cochrane-anaesthesia. suite.dk/
4. Eddy DM. Principles for making difficult decisions in difficult times. *JAMA* 1994; **271**:1792–8.
5. The Infinite List of Systematic Reviews in Anaesthesia and Analgesia. http://www.hcuge.ch/anesthesie/anglais/evidence/arevusyst.htm

For further information and a list of systematic reviews go to http://www. evidbasedanaesth.com

Part I
Evidence-based medicine, randomised trials, and systematic reviews

1: Is evidence-based medicine still an option?

NEVILLE W GOODMAN

"What is the true value of knowledge? That it makes our ignorance more precise."
Anne Michaels. *Fugitive pieces*. London: Bloomsbury, 1998.

"The basic error of EBM is quite simple. It is that epidemiological data do not provide the information necessary to treat individual patients. The error is intractable and intrinsic to the methodological nature of epidemiology, and no amount of statistical jiggery-pokery with huge data sets can make any difference."

Bruce Charlton[1]

Patients are not all the same

About 10 years after the term "evidence-based medicine" was first used, an editorial written by enthusiasts[2] included this statement: "The notion that decisions may vary from circumstance to circumstance, and from patient to patient with the same circumstances, has received increasing attention. But achieving the right balance among the factors that can affect a decision is not necessarily easy". This summarises what is wrong with evidence-based medicine. Not only is what they say true, but critics of evidence-based medicine have been saying it for the whole of the 10 years, and have been ignored. The editorialists ended by suggesting that the term "evidence-based medicine" be replaced by "research enhanced health care", but does that imply that there is some sort of health care that is not research enhanced, and, if so, who would profess to practise it? There are some, it seems, who are unwilling to accept that medicine can be an infuriatingly complicated activity.

Medicine based on evidence is not EBM:
the meaning of "evidence"

In the chapter that introduced the first edition of this book,[3] I distinguished between medicine based on evidence and Evidence-Based Medicine. The capital letters were intentional, and allow the abbreviation EBM. EBM relies mainly on randomised controlled trials (assessed explicitly and strictly), meta-analyses, and megatrials. Although we know that proper evidence is lacking in many fields of health care, nobody argues against medicine that is based on evidence. But EBM is a conceit: it appropriates the word "evidence" placing its own specific meaning on it, and thereby puts critics of EBM – who are presumed to object to the use of evidence at all – at a disadvantage. It is in the meaning of evidence that the disagreements and criticisms lie, and they have not yet been resolved: the evidence of EBM is based in clinical epidemiology, which, as Charlton (see above) drew out[4,5] from the ideas of Feinstein[6,7] among others,[8] is not a sound foundation for the treatment of individual patients.

My own syntheses of these ideas, in detail and fully referenced, are in Chapter 1 of the first edition,[3] and also in a subsequent essay.[9] The arguments from that essay were then developed further,[10] and they still stand. What little counter-criticism there was[11] suffered the problem common to many attempted refutations: getting trapped in the rhetorical bind of using the word "evidence" in the general sense, and not in the specific sense of EBM.

Analysis of EBM: critics ignored

It is instructive to ask colleagues for their views on EBM. Although there are those who are enthusiastically in favour and those who are nihilistically against, there are few who are properly aware of the considered objections to EBM, because in general the enthusiasts do not mention them, nor cite the articles that discuss them. Many medical journals acknowledge some of the difficulties of EBM – in particular, of generalising from randomised controlled trials and of a general lack of evidence – but nonetheless, most journals more or less enthusiastically endorse EBM. The only medical journal that, to my knowledge, has carried any real analysis of EBM is the *Journal of Evaluation in Clinical Practice*, which has now published six thematic issues. The editorial commentary[12] in the latest, sixth issue summarises, by reference to the editorial commentaries in the earlier issues, how the discussion has developed. The main change in EBM has been the acceptance that individual clinicians are unlikely to be able themselves to apply the classical five-step EBM technique, but are likely to have to base their practice on the systematic reviewing of others. There has also been a softening of the authority of the statistical meta-analytic number. But there has been no attempt to refute – that is, to argue logically against – the criticism that this number does not have that authority at all: that meta-analysis and megatrials, inevitably, sacrifice methodological rigour on the altar of statistical precision[5] and cannot therefore be secure bases on which to treat individual patients. As Miles *et al.*[12] write, "the intrinsic and extrinsic limitations of randomised controlled trials and their meta-analyses were effectively ignored", and "doubts about the utility of EBM were treated by its protagonists ... as simply personal problems of the doubter".

The ignoring of limitations continues in the latest issue. Ghali and Sargious[13] attempt a justification of the development of EBM into providing clinical care pathways for busy physicians. (They title their paper *The evolving paradigm of evidence-based medicine*, despite Couto's[14] scathing ridiculing of the use of the word "paradigm". Couto pointed out that EBM is not a new paradigm; it is a new way of approaching particular clinical problems, which, in its "belief in the supremacy of the results of clinical trials over pathophysiology is irrational". But at least Ghali and Sargious have contributed to the dialogue.) The editorial comment is that "Very disappointingly for us, there is no evidence whatsoever in their article of an explicit appreciation of the scientific and clinical limitations of EBM discussed in outline earlier" – which means earlier in the sixth editorial comment – "and in detail elsewhere" – which is referenced to the five previous issues. The editorialists still see evidence of the "familiar 'we know best' pseudoauthority" and are especially upset by Ghali and Sargoius' conclusion that "this new and improved brand of EBM ... will ultimately be central to the maintenance of professionalism in medicine".

The *Journal of Evaluation in Clinical Practice* has carried analysis of EBM, but there has been no real debate about EBM. Debate implies two sides and, as Buetow[15] points out, with a few exceptions the protagonists have "isolated their critics by effectively avoiding them". A good example of this is the Cochrane review of the use of albumin (Chapter 7).[16] Horsey[17] documents the difficulties he had trying to challenge the validity of the review. Swales[18] lamented the complete denial by the review's authors of any "evidence" from the critics because it was not the reviewers' sort of evidence. Horsey worried that the real harm was being done to the Cochrane Collaboration itself by the stubborn refusal of the reviewers to accept they may have been wrong and he comments that it calls into question all the other meta-analyses.

But now we have come full circle: it did not need the albumin review to define the problems of meta-analysis. Feinstein, Charlton, and others have repeatedly (and to me persuasively) explained how meta-analysis is a limited technique, used largely by non-clinical epidemiologists and statisticians. It is another factor of which to take account when treating individual patients, but it cannot be – by virtue of its methodology – the one and most secure basis for treatment.

I have previously commented[9] that the most widely known handbook of EBM cited no critical references at all. Its second edition[19] does ask, "does providing evidence-based care improve outcome for patients?" and "what are the limitations of EBM?". In answer to the first question, they write that population outcome studies show that patients do better if they receive evidence-based (by which they mean EBM-based) therapies, and they give examples from treatments for heart attacks and strokes. But their comparison is of patients who receive these therapies and patients who don't. That is not the question. The true question is whether the process of EBM, as opposed to some other process of drawing conclusions from properly considered available evidence, was necessary to the patients receiving those therapies. Also, it must be true that some meta-analyses will provide a secure clinical answer, because the patients are sufficiently alike in their disease and their response to treatment that generalisation is robust. Given the methodology of meta-analysis and the usual lack of clinical experience of many of the meta-analysts, this is likely to be a matter of luck rather than of scientific consideration. But even if a meta-analytic result is shown to be clinically robust, one cannot then draw conclusions about the robustness of meta-analysis in all circumstances.

The main reference they cite to their second question is a report of a literature search for criticisms of EBM.[20] The authors write that they contacted "experts in the field" (without irony), but although they thank many people well known in EBM circles for comments on earlier versions of the paper, they do not say whether they contacted critical experts as well as supportive experts. They do cite a number of critical papers, although not Feinstein,[6] which many would consider the pivotal one. Their comment on the "basic error" (they cite Charlton[4]) is that biological variability hampers all attempts to extrapolate evidence from basic or applied research to individual patients, and thus the problem is not limited to EBM. However, EBM claims that it *can* be applied to patients, and the problem of variability is no less – in fact it is necessarily more – in a meta-analysis. Straus and McAlister's strongest argument is the circular one – that patients do better if they have been given efficacious treatment. Their counter to EBM being "anti-science" is that there are problems if one uses basic science as a sole basis for treatment.[20]

(Without going into too much detail, the best example of how EBM is anti-science is the application of EBM to alternative medicine.[21] This elevates the idea that clinical trial evidence is the highest form of evidence to ludicrous heights and shows what happens when observations are made outside contextual scientific knowledge. This activity can be done only by people who do not have that knowledge, or who are unable to understand its implications. There are indeed problems if basic science alone is used to treat patients, but from the knowledge of basic science one can formulate properly grounded and clinically testable hypotheses. Unfortunately, the methods of EBM are now being used to provide answers to questions in science.[22,23]

Answers to properly formulated scientific questions will come only from good science.[24] If the science is not yet good enough to provide answers, then we shall have to remain ignorant until it is good enough.)

A systematic review of the evidence

EBM has done some valuable things for medicine. There is no longer any place for physicians who rely completely on what they learned in medical school many years before, whose sole authority was themselves and their experience, and whose only explanation for choice of treatment was "clinical freedom". EBM has made the idea of appraising evidence more familiar to clinicians, and it has enabled easier access to research findings. There are now databases available, and more being planned, for anyone wishing to know what has been published on a subject. Before declaring that there was plenty that had been published "supportive" of EBM, and that "critical" commentaries had not been answered, I needed to do a systematic search myself for anything "counter-critical" that I had missed.

Firstly, however, I thought I would contact one of the well known proponents of EBM by email. I asked if they knew of my challenge to EBM[9] and, more specifically, if they knew of any essay that argued logically against Feinstein's views, but I received no answer to either question.

In early September 2002, I searched Medline (Winspirs) 1999–2002 (August week 2). Searching on "evidence-based medicine" in the title (limited to English language and human studies) produced 486 records. A total of 115 of these were from one series in emergency medicine, which left 371. There are allowable qualifiers for "evidence-based medicine", and there are the universal limiters such as "review", but applying these removed critical papers from the retrieved list. Rejecting papers that, inferring from their titles and abstracts, were also clinical reports left 67 possible papers*. The indexing of clinical trials in medical databases is not perfect, but it is much better than the indexing of papers that are not standard clinical trials: some familiar critical papers were not among the 67.

Thirty-seven papers had abstracts on Medline; I had to obtain copies of the other 30. From this material, it was clear that non-research papers with "evidence-based medicine" in their titles were mostly recipes of how to do EBM, editorials or commentary articles supportive or openly enthusiastic about EBM, or articles critical of it. There were no counter-critical papers. Supportive papers often acknowledged the difficulties of randomised controlled trials, but none commented on the flaw of basing individual treatments on the result of meta-analysis. The "basic error" remains.

It is possible that there was a refutation in one of the abstracted supportive papers, but that this was not mentioned in the abstract. However, knowing how many critical papers there are, and that the commonest criticism is the "basic error", I think it unlikely that authors would omit such an important point. Nor do I think a sound refutation will have been written in another language.

It is not difficult to see why EBM is popular: it is "common sense" (from a supporter);[11] it is "an approach that is intuitively reasonable" (from a critic);[25] "one cannot be 'against' evidence-based medicine because that would imply that one was anti-evidence and thus logically in favour of no evidence" (a critic).[26] Common sense and intuition have been deceived by rhetoric.

Meanwhile, the arguments of the protagonists continue to be circular: "The power of the evidence-based approach has been enhanced in recent years by the development of the techniques of systematic review and meta-analysis. While this approach has its critics, we would all want the best available evidence used in making decisions about our care if we got sick".[27] This begs the question: is meta-analysis the best available evidence?

The new authority of EBM

The irony is that EBM was presumed better than the old authoritarian "paradigm". Yet, by its refusal to acknowledge criticism, the EBM movement has become the new authoritarian. They suggest that being a member of the Cochrane Collaboration is a mark of validity as an expert source, making that person's medical advice authoritative rather than authoritarian.[19] They clearly believe that they are right, and treat critics with the tired disdain that a persistent flat-earther might receive. It is not only doctors who wonder about the religious overtones of EBM. When a journalist asked[28] one of the major influences in the Cochrane Collaboration if there was "a faintly evangelical feel to the collaboration", he received the reply, "Yes, I think that many of the people involved actually do feel that way".

This is not good for medicine. It is not as if the EBM proponents themselves seem to have much faith in clinical research. Haynes[29] wrote that "We're simply going through an evolutionary phase in testing interventions" and, in an editorial[30] about quality scoring of clinical trials, the authors expressed "serious doubts [about] the validity of current clinical research". We should wait for a later stage of evolution before dictating to clinicians the right way to treat patients.

Why don't the EBM proponents at least cite some of the critical papers, acknowledge the disagreement, and ask readers to make up their own minds? That would be the honest approach: more scientific and less dogmatic. The proponent of EBM whom I contacted offered this view of the basic error: "The arguments used by Feinstein and his colleagues are basically that evidence derived from groups, based on probabilities, cannot be directly applied to decisions about individuals. We disagree with this position, which is based on a notion of absolute truth, rather than relative (probabilistic) truth".

This is not an argument; it is a restatement of the position. I do not understand their point about absolute and relative truth but I was given no chance to explore this further because their correspondence ended: "... philosophically, if you are in the Feinstein camp, we're miles apart", and they explicitly refused to respond to any further contact.

EBM is the new authoritarianism.

Is EBM an option?

EBM is an option: "Meta-analyses are systematic reviews ... performed when available evidence is inconclusive. Thus, they should be considered guides to decision making in the face of uncertainty, and their conclusions should be interpreted with caution".[31] Pronovost *et al.*, in reply to my prompting,[32] though they did not counter the "basic error", believe "EBM is a set of tools to assist providers in caring for patients". Assistance is fine; insistence is not. There should be no special authority granted to EBM, not least because of the large areas of medicine in which there is not, nor likely to be, much or any evidence in the near future. The statistic produced by meta-analysis may be appropriate to some patients in some conditions. The importance of that statistic in EBM decisions has been reduced as EBM has developed,[2] but as more and more factors are admitted to medical decisions one starts to wonder in what way "evidence-based medicine" differs from what we used to know as "medicine". (Welsby[33] points out that EBM guidelines used to be known as "textbooks".) EBM becomes nothing special, and risks causing difficulties because the specific acceptable reasons for acting contrary to evidence are not well articulated,[8] and probably cannot be: "the evidence cannot tell us when it is best to ignore the evidence".

Formal systematic review is easier and more appropriate in some specialties than in others.[34–37] Even in those specialties where EBM is most followed, it may be applied to evidence produced from asking the wrong questions.[38]

Swales[39] wrote, "Although advocates of EBM acknowledge the contribution of all forms of evidence, the differential value attached to different sources has led to naive and simplistic attempts to omit the traditional processes of interpretation, synthesis and extrapolation and to draw wide-ranging conclusions from trial data without adequate scientific discussion". My conclusion paraphrases and is an extension of this, and repeats the concluding sentences of an earlier essay.[10] The sort of EBM that is of value is the one where evidence has no special meaning, and where "evidence-based" can be tacked on as a prefix to every topic, every paper and every journal title. Then we can drop the prefix, and get back to the vexed, infuriating, complicated, value laden, rewarding activity that is clinical medicine.

Acknowledgement

I should like to thank Bruce Charlton for his many helpful comments.

References

1. Charlton BG. Book review of evidence-based medicine. *J Eval Clin Pract* 1997;**3**:169–72.
2. Haynes RB, Devereaux PJ, Guyatt GH. Physicians' and patients' choices in evidence based health practice. *BMJ* 2002;**324**:1350.
3. Goodman NW. Evidence based medicine: cautions before using. In: Tramèr M, editor. *Evidence based resource in anaesthesia and analgesia*. London: BMJ Books, 2000:3–25.
4. Charlton BG. Restoring the balance: evidence-based medicine put in its place. *J Eval Clin Pract* 1997;**3**:87–98.
5. Charlton BG. The scope and nature of epidemiology. *J Clin Epidemiol* 1996;**49**:623–6.
6. Feinstein AR. Clinical judgement revisited: the distraction of quantitative models. *Ann Int Med* 1994;**120**:799–805.
7. Feinstein AR, Horwitz RI. Problems in the "Evidence" of "Evidence-based Medicine". *Am J Med* 1997;**103**:529–35.
8. Tonelli MR. The philosophical limits of evidence-based medicine. *Acad Med* 1998;**73**:1234–40.
9. Goodman NW. Who will challenge evidence-based medicine? *J Roy Coll Phys Lond* 1999;**33**:249–51.
10. Goodman NW. In my view … Criticizing evidence-based medicine. *Thyroid* 2000;**10**:157–60.
11. Dent THS. Challenging evidence-based medicine [letter]. *J Roy Coll Phys Lond* 1999;**33**:484–5.
12. Miles A, Grey J, Polychronis A, Melchiorri C. Critical advances in the evaluation and development of clinical care. *J Eval Clin Pract* 2002;**8**:87–102.
13. Ghali WA, Sargious PM. The evolving paradigm of evidence-based medicine. *J Eval Clin Pract* 2002;**8**:109–12.
14. Couto JS. Evidence-based medicine: a Kuhnian perspective of a transvestite non-theory. *J Eval Clin Pract* 1999;**4**:267–75.
15. Buetow S. Beyond evidence-based medicine: bridge-building a medicine of meaning. *J Eval Clin Pract* 2002;**8**:103–8.
16. Cochrane Injuries Group Albumin Reviewers. Human albumin administration in critically ill patients: systematic review of randomised controlled trials. *BMJ* 1998;**317**:235–40.
17. Horsey PJ. The Cochrane 1998 Albumin Review – not all it was cracked up to be. *EJA* 2002;**19**:701–4.
18. Swales JD. The troublesome search for evidence: three cultures in need of integration. *J Roy Soc Med* 2000;**93**:402–7.

19. Sackett DL, Straus SE, Richardson WS, Rosenberg W, Haynes RB. *Evidence based medicine. How to practice and teach EBM.* 2nd ed. New York: Churchill Livingstone, 2001.
20. Straus SE, McAlister FA. Evidence-based medicine: a commentary on common criticisms. *Can Med Ass J* 2000;**163**:837–41.
21. Charlton BG. Randomised trials in alternative/complementary medicine. *Q J Med* 2002;**95**:643–5.
22. Pandit JJ. The variable effect of low-dose volatile anaesthetics on the acute ventilatory response to hypoxia in humans: a quantitative review. *Anaesthesia* 2002;**57**:632–43.
23. Sandercock P, Roberts I. Systematic reviews of animal experiments. *Lancet* 2002;**360**:586.
24. Goodman NW. Knowledge is not measured by the tools of evidence-based medicine. *Anaesthesia* 2002;**57**:1041.
25. Laupacis A. The future of evidence-based medicine. *Can J Clin Pharmacol* 2001;**8** (Suppl. A):6A–9A.
26. Glatstein E. Of scientific physicians and evidence-based medicine. *Int J Radiat Oncol Biol Phys* 2001;**49**:619–21.
27. Davidoff F. In the teeth of the evidence: the curious case of evidence-based medicine. *Mt Sinai J Med* 1999;**66**:75–83.
28. Watts G. Evidence-based medicine. Faith, hope and clarity. *Health Serv J* 1999;**109** (Suppl.):6–7.
29. Haynes B. Can it work? Does it work? Is it worth it? *BMJ* 1999;**319**:652–3.
30. Ioannidis JPA, Lau J. Can quality of clinical trials and meta-analyses be quantified? *Lancet* 1998;**352**:590–1.
31. Lalwani SI, Olive DL. Problems with evidence-based medicine. *J Am Assoc Gynecol Laparosc* 1999;**6**:237–40.
32. Goodman NW. Evidence-based medicine needs proper critical review. *Anesth Analg* 2002;**95**:1817.
33. Welsby PD. Reductionism in medicine: some thoughts on medical education from the clinical front line. *J Eval Clin Pract* 1999;**5**:125–31.
34. Helgason CM, Jobe TH. Causal interactions, fuzzy sets and cerebrovascular "accident": the limits of evidence-based medicine and the advent of complexity-based medicine. *Neuroepidemiology* 1999;**18**:64–74.
35. Saver JL, Kalafut M. Combination therapies and the theoretical limits of evidence-based medicine. *Neuroepidemiology* 2001;**20**:57–64.
36. Williams DDR, Garner J. The case against "the evidence": a different perspective on evidence-based medicine. *Br J Psychiat* 2002;**180**:8–12.
37. Horan BF. Evidence-based medicine and anaesthesia: uneasy bedfellows? *Anaesth Int Care* 1997;**25**:679–85.
38. Julian DG, Norris RM. Myocardial infarction: is evidence-based medicine the best? *Lancet* 2002;**359**:1515–6.
39. Swales JD. Evidence-based medicine and hypertension. *J Hypertens* 1999;**17**:1511–6.

*The material available on Medline (Winspirs) from the 67 retrieved papers is available from the author by email (Nev.W.Goodman@bris.ac.uk).

2: Why do we need large randomised trials in anaesthesia and analgesia?

PAUL S MYLES

Introduction

Clinical practice should be guided by medical research. Each type of research – basic sciences, animal, clinical, epidemiological, and others – provides different elements. All of them are important, can be complementary, and have a role in evidence-based practice. But it is the randomised controlled clinical trial that provides the most reliable information about the efficacy of a proposed treatment in clinical practice.[1-5] Yet most clinical trials do not cause a change in practice; this suggests either that their results are unreliable or that such trials are irrelevant to clinical practice. The purpose of this chapter is to explain why investigation of moderate treatment effects on important outcomes is best done using large, simple, randomised trials.

Reliability, or precision, is important to clinicians because we want to be able to estimate the probable effect of any new treatment and determine whether this would be clinically important in any particular circumstance. If uncertainty exists then we are likely to defer a change in practice until further confirmatory evidence appears.[6-8] Unfortunately, there is often a substantial amount of conflicting information in the literature that further confuses the issue, and this can hinder interest and uptake of evidence-based medicine (EBM) by practising clinicians. A trial is more likely to be influential if it reflects standard clinical practice.[1-4] Clinicians need to consider evidence from clinical trials; this is helped when such trials have been conducted in a real-world setting, studying typical patients. This is often not the case, with interested researchers studying selected groups of patients in specialised settings.[9-12] Furthermore, anaesthesia research frequently uses surrogate end points – biochemical markers, urine flow, myocardial ischaemia, cerebral blood flow, recovery times, and so on – which are of questionable significance and often have no convincing relation to patient outcome.[2,9,13,14]

These two features – reliability and relevance – could be addressed by studying every single patient from around the world with any particular condition of interest. Such a large trial would be a massive undertaking and is beyond the realms of practicality and funding. Do we need to study all patients? If not, how large does a trial need to be in order to be feasible but not sacrifice reliability? Are meta-analyses of small trials the answer? Do we need to conduct a randomised trial, or could we collect routine clinical data that would still enable us to reliably identify effective treatments?

Large observational studies can be misleading.[15] A striking example is hormone replacement therapy: despite multiple cohort studies over many years suggesting benefits, the recent Women's Health Initiative study,[16] a large trial in more than 16 000 women, found that oestrogen–progesterone replacement leads to excess stroke, myocardial infarction, breast cancer, and pulmonary embolism. Examples can also be found in perioperative medicine: there have been numerous observational studies (and some small trials) illustrating a beneficial effect of regional blockade on outcome after major surgery, but two recent large trials did not find a significant difference when comparing combined epidural–general anaesthesia with general anaesthesia alone.[17,18] A recent cohort study investigated the risks and benefits of aspirin after coronary bypass surgery in 5065 patients and found a significant reduction in mortality with aspirin (1·3% v 4·0%, P < 0·001).[19] Such an effect, if it were real, would be of great importance and challenges the widespread practice of stopping aspirin perioperatively. But this was not a randomised trial; there could be other explanations for the results,[20] and so it is unlikely to have a major impact on clinical practice until a large trial confirms its main findings.

Non-randomised studies are commonly biased.[15,21] We know that outcome after surgery is dependent on many factors, and so a new treatment being studied may have a spurious association with a good outcome that is unrelated to any true effect. Random allocation to treatment groups accounts for many of these:

- selection bias, in allocating patients to each treatment group
- treatment bias, when considering additional treatments during the study
- measurement and detection bias, in recording outcomes, and so on.

But random allocation to treatment groups does not account for all forms of bias. An imbalance in prognostic factors – a situation known as confounding – may still exist, and this is particularly likely if such factors have a potent effect on outcome.[1-4,22] A large randomised trial will equalise all such factors, both known and unknown, between groups.[1-4,12] This is one of the major strengths of large trials.

Accurate reporting of trials is necessary in order to identify those that may not have acceptable levels of bias control. The CONSORT statement includes a list of criteria used to identify the most important features of a reliable trial;[23] it is anticipated that improvement in the quality of reporting clinical trials should facilitate access to best evidence and improve health care.

An observed difference between groups might not be a true difference but a chance finding (a type I, or α error). If no significant difference is found it could be that the study was not large enough to detect a true difference, and so its conclusion may be incorrect (a type II, or β error). A study's power describes the likelihood of being able to detect a true difference between groups. A key requirement for maximising study power is to study enough patients, and so an adequate sample size must be determined before commencing a study (Table 2.1).

For these reasons, evidence from small trials can be unreliable because they provide imprecise estimates of effect, as illustrated by their wide confidence intervals.[1-4,6,7,12] For example, a randomised trial of 477 patients concluded that the inotropic drug vesnarinone reduced mortality in patients with heart failure (26 v 50 patients, P = 0·003).[24] A large trial (n = 3833) subsequently found a dose-dependent *increased* mortality with vesnarinone (292 v 242 deaths, P = 0·02).[25] Conversely, small trials had previously suggested that beta-blockers may be harmful in patients with severe heart failure, yet a recent large trial has shown these drugs to have a clear benefit in this group of patients.[26] Many small trials have found that growth hormone can improve a variety of surrogate outcomes, such as the catabolic response to injury, surgery, and sepsis. However, the effect of high doses of growth hormone on outcome in critically ill adults was not known. A large European trial found a twofold increase in hospital mortality in the patients who received growth hormone (P < 0·001).[27] Interestingly, a large trial of intensive glucose control with insulin has recently been shown to provide a clear benefit in such patients (see below).[28]

Inconsistent findings are more likely when the evidence base is limited to small trials.[29,30] Some characteristics of the trial population (selective recruitment, specialised clinical environment, compliance to treatment, and so on) may mean that a treatment effect is inflated or missed.[7,12] Large trials provide precise estimates of effect; small trials cannot.

A meta-analysis of all relevant trials will provide least-biased estimates, but this has some potential weaknesses,[14,22,24,25,30-32] particularly if limited to small trials.[4,29-32] Meta-analyses sometimes give conflicting results when compared with large trials.[30-32] For example, Lelorier and colleagues found that 35% of the outcomes of

Table 2.1 Sample size: how many patients should be studied? The relationship between incidence, absolute risk reduction, effect size, and the likelihood of detecting a true difference (study power)

Incidence in current practice (control group) (%)	Incidence in the intervention group (%)	Absolute risk reduction*	Effect size*	Sample size† 80% power (β error 0·2)	Sample size† 90% power (β error 0·1)
50	40	0·1	0·2	1040	1280
	25	0·25	0·5	160	190
	10	0·4	0·8	50	62
20	16	0·04	0·2	3900	4800
	10	0·1	0·5	530	660
	8	0·12	0·8	350	430
10	8	0·02	0·2	8600	10 600
	5	0·05	0·5	1200	1440
	2	0·08	0·8	370	450
5	4	0·01	0·2	18 000	22 300
	2·5	0·025	0·5	2400	3000
	1	0·04	0·8	760	840

*The absolute risk reduction and effect size (treatment effect) are described as proportions, whereby 0·1 ≡ 10%
†Design V1·0 statistical software

12 large trials were not predicted by meta-analyses published previously.[31] A frequently cited example is the effect of magnesium sulphate on outcome in patients with acute myocardial infarction.[30-34] Nevertheless, if there are no large trials available then a meta-analysis of all available trials remains the best level of evidence.

Postoperative major morbidity and death are uncommon and new treatments are likely to have only a moderate effect on outcome. Dickinson and colleagues recently identified 203 small trials in head injury, which had reported on a total of 16–613 patients.[7] The average number of patients in each trial was 82. No trials were large enough to detect reliably a 5% absolute risk reduction in death or disability. Only 4% were large enough to detect an absolute risk reduction of 10%. They concluded that currently available trials are too small to be able to detect or refute clinically important benefits or risks.[7] It is pertinent to bear in mind that the average treatment effect of new interventions in "positive" trials is about 20% (that is, an effect size of 0·2). Such effects are frequently "clouded" by other factors – these are known as systematic and random errors. Systematic error, or bias, is best dealt with by attention to study design and conduct, the most important step being random allocation to treatment groups. Random error includes measurement imprecision and biological variation – "background noise". These sources of error are often larger than the effect of interest.[1-4] Because most improvements in perioperative medicine are incremental, large numbers of patients need to be studied in order to have the power to detect a clinically significant difference.[3,35] An increase in sample size will reduce random error, but will not reduce bias.

Large trials are usually multicentred, and sometimes multinational, to maximise recruitment and enable early conclusion.[1,2] This provides a broad range of settings and offers an opportunity to identify other patient, clinician, and institutional factors that may influence outcome. As stated above, these extraneous, potentially confounding factors are more likely to be balanced between groups in large trials.[1,2,12,22,36] Large trials are therefore less biased and are more reliable.[1,2,12,22,35,36] What is a large trial? This depends on the clinical scenario, but it could be defined as a trial in 1000 patients or more with adequate power (> 80%) to detect a true difference for an important outcome.[2,30,31] Yet, adverse outcomes after surgery are rare. For example, the incidence of stroke, renal failure, or death after coronary artery surgery is mostly less than 4%. Study power is determined by the number of trial events, and so power can be increased by focusing on high-risk patients and/or by using a combined end point.[36] In each case there will be more outcome events in the trial, and the likelihood of detecting a difference, if it exists, will be increased – fewer patients need to be studied in a high-risk population. Study power is also affected by the size of the treatment effect being investigated – a large effect can be detected with a smaller sample size. These features are illustrated in Table 2.1.

In order to be feasible, large trials should have straightforward requirements.[1-3] The use of simply defined interventions and outcome assessments can assist the conduct of large trials; this will also support their uptake into clinical practice because stringent experimental conditions might otherwise preclude applicability to standard practice. Large, simple trials reflect standard practice and are sometimes called "effectiveness" trials.[1,5,12,35] They are reliable and relevant.

There have been some excellent examples of large trials in perioperative medicine[18,28,37-43] (see Table 2.2). Van den Berghe and colleagues, in a large trial of 1548 critical care patients, compared an intensive insulin regimen with conventional treatment.[28] They found that intensive insulin therapy reduced mortality during intensive care from 8·0% with conventional treatment to 4·6% (P < 0·04). There was also a beneficial effect on deaths due to multi-organ failure, sepsis, acute renal failure, red-cell transfusions, polyneuropathy, and need for prolonged mechanical ventilation and intensive care.[28] This trial has had an immediate effect on clinical practice throughout the world.

Large trials are not foolproof, nor are they the exclusive currency of EBM.[5,8,44] Their main strength lies in the ability to detect small-to-moderate treatment effects, but they may overlook a specific effect, or subgroup, that could be identified by a small trial with more tightly controlled intervention in a uniform group of patients. In addition, small trials have a particular strength in medical research: studying surrogate end points to gain mechanistic insight into why an outcome has occurred, helping "build a case" of cause and effect.[4,33] Dose–response relationships, drug interaction (or combinations), and effects on patients with complex or multisystem disease can be ascertained. Similarly, large observational cohort studies have a role in evidence-based practice. Concato and colleagues have shown that rigorous observational studies with contemporaneous controls provide reliable evidence in some circumstances.[45] Even so, MacMahon and Collins have outlined many of the weaknesses of observational studies.[15] Their strengths lie in detecting rare events, such as side effects of treatment, and identifying possible interventions that ought to be tested with a large trial.

Some have argued that large trials can be misleading, particularly when they represent select populations.[11] It is true that generalisation from trials to clinical practice may be limited – the relevance argument – but the solution should be to design large trials that reflect real-world practice. Alternative approaches have been suggested,[11] but these cannot account for bias and confounding.[20] Large trials also provide an opportunity to identify subgroups of interest and mechanistic explanations of effect.

EBM teaches clinicians to identify reliable studies that are relevant to a condition of interest. A classification of studies, based on reliability

Table 2.2 Examples of large, randomised trials in perioperative medicine

Reference	Main findings	Sample size (n)
Kurz et al. 1996[37]	Maintenance of normothermia during colorectal surgery reduces wound infection and length of hospital stay	200
Greif et al. 2000[38]	Supplemental oxygen ($FiO_2 > 0.8$) reduces wound infection after colorectal surgery	500
PEP Trial Group 2000[39]	Low-dose aspirin reduces venous thrombosis and pulmonary embolism after hip surgery	14 244
ARDS Network 2000[40]	In patients with acute lung injury or acute respiratory distress syndrome, mechanical ventilation with a lower tidal volume decreases mortality and duration of mechanical ventilation	861
Bernard et al. 2001[41]	Treatment with activated protein C reduces mortality in patients with severe sepsis	1690
van den Berghe et al. 2001[28]	Intensive insulin therapy for hyperglycaemia reduces mortality and major morbidity in critically ill patients	1548
Magpie Trial Group 2002[42]	Magnesium halves the risk of eclampsia, and probably reduces the risk of maternal death	10 141
Rigg et al. 2002[18]	Combined general anaesthesia and regional block does not reduce mortality or major morbidity in high-risk patients undergoing major abdominal surgery	915
Johnson et al. 2002[43]	When compared with aspirin alone, long-term combined warfarin–aspirin anticoagulation increases mortality and morbidity after peripheral vascular surgery	831

(levels of evidence), places trials and meta-analyses of trials in top position. But the interpretation of published evidence ought to go beyond categorising levels of evidence according to a hierarchical scale, to consider additional sources of information, such as observational studies and audit,[11,45] and clinical experience. Consistency of an effect provides strong evidence. A key step of EBM, one frequently overlooked by critics of EBM, is to critically appraise the evidence and give consideration to the relevance of a particular clinical situation. This can confirm the applicability, and extent of benefit, to actual patients of interest. Clear thinking, clinical judgement, and perspective are important elements of evidence-based practice.

The introduction to this chapter identified several types of research used to guide clinical practice. In most cases, clinicians aim to make a diagnosis, and choose a treatment that is most likely to be effective. This decision making is often influenced by cost and resource considerations. Large trials rightly deserve the mantle of "gold standard" in providing evidence of effectiveness, because they provide reliable, relevant information to guide our practice.

References

1. Yusuf S, Collins R, Peto R. Why do we need some large, simple randomized trials? *Stat Med* 1984;**3**:409–20.
2. Myles PS. Why we need large randomised studies in anaesthesia. *Br J Anaesth* 1999;**83**:833–4.
3. Peto R, Baigent C. Trials: the next 50 years. Large scale randomised evidence of moderate benefits. *BMJ* 1998;**317**:1170–1.
4. Collins R, MacMahon S. Reliable assessment of the effects of treatment on mortality and major morbidity, I: clinical trials. *Lancet* 2001;**357**:373–80.
5. Rigg JRA, Jamrozik K, Myles PS. Evidence-based methods to improve anaesthesia and intensive care. *Curr Opin Anaesthesiol* 1999;**12**:221–7.
6. Kelly MJU, Wadsworth J. What price inconclusive clinical trials? *Ann R Coll Surg Eng* 1993;**75**:145–6.
7. Dickinson K, Bunn F, Wentz R, Edwards P, Roberts I. Size and quality of randomised controlled trials in head injury: review of published studies. *BMJ* 2000;**320**:1308–11.
8. Sniderman AD. Clinical trials, consensus conferences, and clinical practice. *Lancet* 1999;**354**:327–30.
9. Horan B. Evidence based medicine and anaesthesia: uneasy bedfellows? *Anaesth Intensive Care* 1997;**25**:679–85.
10. Goodman NW. Anaesthesia and evidence-based medicine. *Anaesthesia* 1998;**53**:353–68.
11. Charlton BG. The future of clinical research: from megatrials towards methodological rigour and representative sampling. *J Eval Clin Pract* 1996;**2**:159–69.
12. McPeek B. Inference, generalizability, and a major change in anesthetic practice. *Anesthesiology* 1987;**66**:723–4.
13. Fisher DM. Surrogate outcomes: meaningful not! *Anesthesiology* 1999;**90**:355–6.
14. Lee A, Lum ME. Measuring anaesthetic outcomes. *Anaesth Intensive Care* 1996;**24**:685–93.
15. MacMahon S, Collins R. Reliable assessment of the effects of treatment on mortality and major morbidity, II: observational studies. *Lancet* 2001;**357**:455–62.
16. Women's Health Initiative Investigators. Risks and benefits of estrogen plus progestin in healthy postmenopausal women: principal results from the Women's Health Initiative randomized controlled trial. *JAMA* 2002;**288**:321–33.

17. Park WY, Thompson JS, Lee KK. Effect of epidural anesthesia and analgesia on perioperative outcome: a randomized, controlled Veterans Affairs cooperative study. *Ann Surg* 2001;**234**:560–71.
18. Rigg JRA, Jamrozik K, Myles PS, *et al.* Epidural anaesthesia and analgesia and outcome of major surgery: a randomised trial. *Lancet* 2002;**359**:1276–82.
19. Mangano DT, Multicenter Study of Perioperative Ischemia Research Group. Aspirin and mortality from coronary bypass surgery. *N Engl J Med* 2002;**347**:1309–17.
20. Datta M. You cannot exclude the explanation you have not considered. *Lancet* 1993;**342**:345–7.
21. Sacks H, Chalmers TC, Smith H Jr. Randomized versus historical controls for clinical trials. *Am J Med* 1982;**72**:233–40.
22. Rothman KJ. Epidemiologic methods in clinical trials. *Cancer* 1977;**39**:S1771–5.
23. Moher D, Schulz KF, Altman DG, for the CONSORT Group. The CONSORT statement: revised recommendations for improving the quality of reports of parallel-group randomised trials. *Lancet* 2001;**357**:1191–4.
24. Feldman AM, Bristow MR, Parmley WW, *et al.* Effects of vesnarinone on morbidity and mortality in patients with heart failure. Vesnarinone Study Group. *N Engl J Med* 1993;**329**:149–55.
25. Cohn JN, Goldstein SO, Greenberg BH, *et al.* A dose-dependent increase in mortality with vesnarinone among patients with severe heart failure. Vesnarinone Trial Investigators. *N Engl J Med* 1998;**339**:1810–6.
26. Packer M, Coats AJ, Fowler MB, *et al.* Effect of carvedilol on survival in severe chronic heart failure. *N Engl J Med* 2001;**344**:1651–8.
27. Takala J, Ruokonen E, Webster NR, *et al.* Increased mortality associated with growth hormone treatment in critically ill adults. *N Engl J Med* 1999;**341**:785–92.
28. van den Berghe G, Wouters P, Weekers F, *et al.* Intensive insulin therapy in the critically ill patients. *N Engl J Med* 2001;**345**:1359–67.
29. Moher D, Jones A, Cook DJ, *et al.* Does quality of reports of randomised trials affect estimates of intervention efficacy reported in meta-analyses? *Lancet* 1998;**352**:609–13.
30. Cappelleri JC, Ioannidis JPA, Schmid CH, *et al.* Large trials vs meta-analysis of smaller trials: how do their results compare? *JAMA* 1996;**276**:1332–8.
31. LeLoerier J, Gregoire G, Benhaddad A, Lapierre J, Derderian Fl. Discrepancies between meta-analyses and subsequent large randomized, controlled trials. *N Engl J Med* 1997;**337**:536–42.
32. Egger M, Smith GD. Misleading meta-analysis: lessons learned from "an effective, safe, simple" intervention that wasn't. *BMJ* 1995;**310**:752–4.
33. Woods KL. Mega-trials and management of acute myocardial infarction. *Lancet* 1995;**346**:611–4.
34. Antman EM. Randomized trials of magnesium in acute myocardial infarction: big numbers do not tell the whole story. *Am J Cardiol* 1995;**75**:391–3.
35. Rigg JR, Jamrozik K, Clarke M. How can we demonstrate that new developments in anaesthesia are of real clinical importance? *Anesthesiology* 1997;**86**:1008–11.
36. Ioannidis JPA, Lau J. The impact of high-risk patients on the results of clinical trials. *J Clin Epidemiol* 1997;**50**:1089–98.
37. Kurz A, Sessler DI, Lenhardt R, The Study of Wound Infection and Temperature Group. Perioperative normothermia to reduce the incidence of surgical-wound infection and shorten hospitalization. *N Engl J Med* 1996;**334**:1209–15.
38. Greif R, Akca O, Horn EP, Kurz A, Sessler DI. Supplemental perioperative oxygen to reduce the incidence of surgical-wound infection. Outcomes Research Group. *N Engl J Med* 2000;**342**:161–7.
39. The PEP Trial Collaborative Group. Prevention of pulmonary embolism and deep vein thrombosis with low dose aspirin: Pulmonary Embolism Prevention (PEP) trial. *Lancet* 2000;**355**:1295–302.
40. The Acute Respiratory Distress Syndrome Network. Ventilation with lower tidal volumes as compared with traditional tidal volumes for acute lung injury and the acute respiratory distress syndrome. *N Engl J Med* 2000;**342**:1301–8.
41. Bernard GR, Vincent JL, Laterre PF, *et al.* Efficacy and safety of recombinant human activated protein C for severe sepsis. *N Engl J Med* 2001;**344**:699–709.

42. The Magpie Trial Collaboration Group. Do women with pre-eclampsia, and their babies, benefit from magnesium sulphate? The Magpie Trial: a randomised placebo-controlled trial. *Lancet* 2002;**359**:1877–90.
43. Johnson WC, Williford WO. Benefits, morbidity, and mortality associated with long-term administration of oral anticoagulant therapy to patients with peripheral arterial bypass procedures: a prospective randomized study. *J Vasc Surg* 2002;**35**:413–21.
44. Evidence-based medicine working group. Evidence-based medicine: a new approach to teaching the practice of medicine. *JAMA* 1992;**268**:2420–5.
45. Concato J, Shah N, Horwitz RI. Randomized, controlled trials, observational studies, and the hierarchy of research designs. *N Engl J Med* 2000;**342**:1887–92.

3: Why do we need systematic reviews in anaesthesia and analgesia?

R ANDREW MOORE

We need systematic reviews in anaesthesia and analgesia for a number of reasons: to tell us what we do not know; to tell us what we do know, and be sure of it; and, perhaps, most importantly, to inform on what are the research questions and study designs for the future. For the avoidance of doubt, none of these statements makes a claim that systematic reviews, or randomised trials, are the only way we move forward, and there are circumstances in which neither systematic reviews nor randomised trials are what we need.

The ethical dimension dominates all these. Should any new study be undertaken without a full appreciation about what is already known? No new trial should be done without a search for extant systematic reviews, or, if they are not available, a new systematic review or at least a systematic search should be done. This used to be a laborious and complicated business. But now we have online searching of electronic databases available to all, and the Cochrane Library has a database of over 250 000 controlled trials and many thousands of reviews (Chapter 11).

To tell us what we do not know

The job of a systematic review is to pull all the nuggets of gold from piles of dross, not to give us one big pile of dross that may or may not have some nuggets in it. What we seek, but unfortunately do not always get, is a good review of good trials (Figure 3.1). A bad review of good trials can at least be repeated to gain more information. A good review of inadequate trials may be helpful, if it identifies trials and problems with them. An inadequate review of inadequate trials may mislead if authors of the review are overenthusiastic about their findings.

The Cochrane Library now has about 1300 reviews published by the Collaboration. Many of them can find little or no evidence in the form of properly conducted randomised trials for that particular topic.

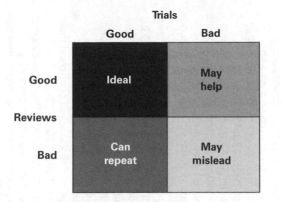

Figure 3.1 Relationship between clinical trials and systematic reviews

Identifying where there is no evidence is an important, though often overlooked, service we get from the Cochrane Collaboration.

To tell us what we do know

Good systematic reviews of good randomised trials can give solid pieces of knowledge, including not only that an intervention works (a statistical result), but how well it works (a clinically relevant result). We need to know what makes a good review to judge how much to trust it.

The key to this is that the review should take steps to avoid known sources of systematic bias (Table 3.1). The most important components for trials of treatment effectiveness are randomisation and blinding. Including non-randomised or open trials may (though not necessarily always) produce results that are completely different from results produced by randomised and double-blind studies. Other known sources of bias include covert duplication and where a study has been done.

If a systematic review is to tell us what we do know, then as well as avoiding bias, there has to be enough information to be certain of a result, and the result has to be expressed in a way we can understand. We also need to know that patients in the review reflect the population in which we want to use the result. These issues deserve a special mention.

Size

Several studies have looked at random chance and clinical trials, reminding us how often and how much chance can affect results. One study actually used dice to mimic clinical trials in stroke prevention.[1]

Table 3.1 Known sources of bias

Source of bias	Effect on treatment efficacy	Size of the effect	References
Randomisation	Increase	Non-randomised studies overestimate treatment effect by 41% with inadequate method, 30% with unclear method	Schultz KF, Chalmers I, Hayes RJ, Altman DG. Empirical evidence of bias: dimensions of methodological quality associated with estimates of treatment effects in controlled trials. *JAMA* 1995;**273**:408–12
Randomisation	Increase	Completely different result between randomised and non-randomised studies	Carroll D, Tramèr M, McQuay H, Nye B, Moore A. Randomization is important in studies with pain outcomes: systematic review of transcutaneous electrical nerve stimulation in acute postoperative pain. *Br J Anaesth* 1996;**77**:798–803
Blinding	Increase	17%	Schultz KF, Chalmers I, Hayes RJ, Altman DG. Empirical evidence of bias: dimensions of methodological quality associated with estimates of treatment effects in controlled trials. *JAMA* 1995;**273**:408–12
Blinding	Increase	Completely different result between blind and non-blind studies	Ernst E, White AR. Acupuncture for back pain: a meta-analysis of randomised controlled trials. *Arch Int Med* 1998;**158**:2235–41
Reporting quality	Increase	About 25%	Khan KS, Daya S, Jadad AR. The importance of quality of primary studies in producing unbiased systematic reviews. *Arch Intern Med* 1996;**156**:661–6
Moher D, Pham B, Jones A, *et al.* Does quality of reports of randomised trials affect estimates of intervention efficacy reported in meta-analyses? *Lancet* 1998;**352**:609–13

(Continued)

Table 3.1 (Continued)

Source of bias	Effect on treatment efficacy	Size of the effect	References
Duplication	Increase	About 20%	Tramèr M, Reynolds DJM, Moore RA, McQuay HJ. Effect of covert duplicate publication on meta-analysis: a case study. *BMJ* 1997;**315**:635–40
Geography	Increase	May be large for some alternative therapies	Vickers A, Goyal N, Harland R, Rees R. Do certain countries produce only positive results? A systematic review of controlled trials. *Control Clin Trial* 1998;**19**:159–66
Size	Increase	Small trials may overestimate treatment effects by about 30%	Moore RA, Tramèr M, Carroll D, Wiffen PJ, McQuay HJ. Quantitative systematic review of topically-applied non-steroidal anti-inflammatory drugs. *BMJ* 1998;**316**:333–8 Moore RA, Gavaghan D, Tramèr MR, Collins SL, McQuay HJ. Size is everything: large amounts of information are needed to overcome random effects in estimating direction and magnitude of treatment effects. *Pain* 1998;**78**:217–20
Statistical	Increase	Not known to any extent, probably modest, but important especially where vote-counting occurs	Smith LA, Oldman AD, McQuay HJ, Moore RA. Teasing apart quality and validity in systematic reviews: an example from acupuncture trials in chronic neck and back pain. *Pain* 2000;**86**:119–32
Validity	Increase	Not known to any extent, probably modest, but important especially where vote-counting occurs	Smith LA, Oldman AD, McQuay HJ, Moore RA. Teasing apart quality and validity in systematic reviews: an example from acupuncture trials in chronic neck and back pain. *Pain* 2000;**86**:119–32

(Continued)

Table 3.1 (Continued)

Source of bias	Effect on treatment efficacy	Size of the effect	References
Language	Increase	Not known to any extent, but may be modest	Egger M, Zellweger-Zähner T, Schneider M, Junker C, Lengeler C, Antes G. Language bias in randomised controlled trials published in English and German. *Lancet* 1997;**350**:326–9
Publication	Increase	Not known to any extent, probably modest, but important especially where there is little evidence	Egger M, Smith GD. Under the meta-scope: potentials and limitations of meta-analysis. In: Tramèr M, ed. *Evidence based resource in anaesthesia and analgesia*. London: BMJ Publications, 2000

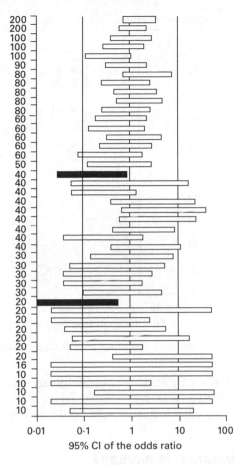

95% CI of the odds ratio

Figure 3.2 Odds ratios for individual "dice" studies, by number in "trial"

If a six was thrown, this was recorded as a death, with any other number recorded as survival. The procedure was repeated for a control group of similar size, ranging from 5 to 100 "patients".

The paper gives the results of all 44 "trials" for 2256 "patients". Since each arm of the trial looks for the throwing of one out of six possibilities for standard dice, we might expect that the rate of events was 16·7% (100/6) in each, with an odds ratio or relative risk of 1. The odds ratios found for individual trials are shown in Figure 3.2. Two trials (20 and 40 "patients" in total) had odds ratios statistically different from 1 – roughly what we would expect by chance.

The variability in individual trial arms is shown in Figure 3.3, which shows the results for all 88 trial arms. The vertical line shows the overall result (16·7%). Larger samples come close to this, but small samples show values as low as zero, and as high as 60%. The overall result, pooling data from all 44 trials, showed that events occurred in 16·0% of

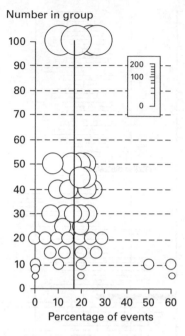

Number in group

Figure 3.3 Percentage of events in each trial arm of "dice" "trials"

treatments and 17·6% of controls (overall mean 16·7%). The overall relative risk was 0·8 (0·5–1·1), but smaller trials, with 30 per group or less, actually came up with a statistically significant result (Table 3.2).

How much information is enough?

While it is relatively easy to demonstrate that inadequate amounts of information can result in erroneous conclusions, the alternative question – how much information do we need to avoid erroneous conclusions? – is more difficult to answer. It depends on a number of things. Two important issues are the size of the effect you are looking at (absolute differences between treatment and control), and how sure you want to be.

A worked example using simulations of acute pain trials[2] gives us some idea. The same 16% event rate as in the dice trials above was used as the rate with controls (because it happens to be what is found with placebo). The example looks at event rates with treatment of 40%, 50%, and 60%, equivalent to numbers-needed-to-treat (NNT) of 4·2, 2·9, and 2·3. The numbers in treatment and placebo groups were each simulated from 25 patients per group (trial size 50) to 500 patients per group (trial size 1000). For each condition, 10 000 trials were simulated and the percentage where the NNT was within ± 0·5 of the true NNT counted.

Table 3.2 Meta-analysis of dice "trials", with sensitivity analysis by size of trial

	No of		Outcome (%) with		Relative risk	NNT
	Trials	Patients	Treatment	Control	(95% CI)	(95% CI)
All trials	44	2256	16·0	17·6	0·8 (0·5 to 1·1)	62 (21 to −67)
Larger trials (> 40 per group)	11	1190	19·5	17·8	1·1 (0·9 to 1·4)	−60 (36 to −16)
Smaller trials (< 40 per group)	33	1066	12·0	17·3	0·7 (0·5 to 0·9)	19 (11 to 98)

CI = confidence interval; NNT = number needed to treat

Table 3.3 Effect of size and magnitude of effect on confidence of treatment effect

	Per cent events with treatment		
	40	**50**	**60**
	4.2	**NNT** **2.9**	**2.3**
Group size			
25	26	37	57
50	28	51	73
100	38	61	88
200	55	81	96
300	63	89	99
400	71	93	99
500	74	95	100

With control the event rate was 16%
NNT = number needed to treat

At least:
50%   within ± 0.5
80%   within ± 0.5
95%   within ± 0.5

The results are shown in Table 3.3. With 1000 patients in a trial where the NNT was 2·3, we could be 100% sure that the NNT measured was within ± 0·5 (1·8–2·8) of the true NNT. In a trial of 50 patients where the NNT was 4·2, only one in four trials would produce an NNT within ± 0·5 (3·7–4·7).

The study also shows that to be certain of the size of the effect (the NNT, say), we need 10 times more information than to know that there is statistical significance.

Not only do we need well conducted trials of robust design and reporting, we also need large amounts of information if the size of a clinical effect is to be accurately assessed. The rule of thumb is that where the difference between control and treatment is small we need very large amounts. Only when the difference is large (an absolute risk increase or decrease of 50%, affecting every second patient) can we be reasonably happy with information from 500 patients or fewer.

When we see differences between trials, or between responses to placebo, the rush is often to try and explain the difference according to some facet of trial design or patient characteristic. Rarely or never is the first, and most sensible, move to ask how likely the difference is to occur just by the random play of chance. One reason for needing systematic reviews is to reduce the effects of random chance.

Outputs

When systematic reviews combine information from many studies in a meta-analysis, the result is often expressed in some statistical form, like an odds ratio or relative risk. Few people understand these, and fewer can use the results expressed in this way. More understand outputs that reflect the therapeutic effort needed to generate one clinically useful result, like the NNT. Even more useful could be the absolute percentage of patients who benefit from treatment.

The following procedure can help when looking at outputs from systematic reviews and meta-analyses:

1. First check on the statistical result
2. If statistically significant, proceed to calculate an NNT. Use the NNT to estimate the *treatment specific therapeutic effort* needed for one outcome to give clinical relevance to the result
3. If this seems sensible, look at what percentage of patients benefit with (or are harmed by) treatment, and use this figure for everyday work because this is immediately clinically relevant every time.

How results are expressed is important, and studies have repeatedly shown that relative risk, and especially relative risk reduction, get doctors more excited. In the first of these studies, David Naylor and colleagues[3] compared clinicians' ratings of therapeutic effectiveness by looking at different endpoints presented as per cent reductions in relative risk, absolute risk, and NNTs. The study was conducted using random allocation of questionnaires using relative data or absolute data, each with NNT, among doctors of various grades at Toronto teaching hospitals. They used an 11-point scale anchored at "no effect" and running from −5 ("harmful") to +5 ("very effective").

Relative presentation consistently showed a tendency to higher scores – that is, the intervention was interpreted as being more effective (Figure 3.4). Where data from a single end point, for any myocardial infarction, were examined, both relative and absolute comparison was scored consistently higher than NNT presentation of the same data. NNT reporting of the same information produced a reduction of about two points in the effectiveness scale, reducing the judgement from quite effective to one of only slight effect. Systematic reviews should use a variety of outputs so that people can understand what the result means, and how they can best use that knowledge.

Patients like ours

A systematic review claimed that mortality and morbidity were decreased with epidural or spinal anaesthesia.[4] The review was exemplary in the way it searched for papers, found additional

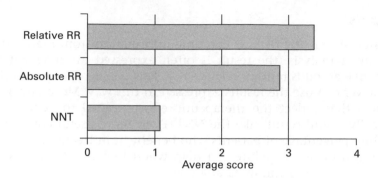

Figure 3.4 Scoring effectiveness on "any myocardial infarction" by method of presentation. NNT = number needed to treat; RR = risk reduction

information, contacted authors, and extracted data. The aim was to find all trials where patients were randomised to neuraxial blockade or not.

There were 141 trials with 9559 patients, and 247 deaths within 30 days, recorded in 35 trials. Most trials had no deaths or, at most, a few deaths. There were nine trials with at least 10 deaths per trial, and these are shown in Figure 3.5. For only three smaller trials was there a large effect of neuraxial blockade, and in these three there was an extraordinarily high death rate with control of over 15%. For six other trials in which the death rate with control was below 15%, the death rates with neuraxial blockade and control were about the same. Over all 141 trials there was a protective effect of neuraxial blockade (NNT 98 to prevent one death). Excluding trials with death rates over 10%, the effect of neuraxial blockade was very small, reducing the death rate from 2·1% in controls who did not receive neuraxial blockade to 1·8% in 136 trials with 94% of the patients.

Why should we exclude trials with death rates above 10% in controls? Because we do not often see death rates that high from surgery, and certainly not the death rates of 15–25% seen in these trials from the early 1980s. These patients are not like ours. In patients who were like ours, with low death rates, there was no effect of anaesthetic technique, as two more recent large randomised studies have confirmed.[5,6] Systematic reviews should reflect patients like ours, or highlight differences in treatment effects in patients with different disease severity.

Setting the research agenda

Systematic reviews are medical archaeology. They tell us about the past, and that past may well be relevant to the present and the future. What was thought of as adequate in the past may well not be

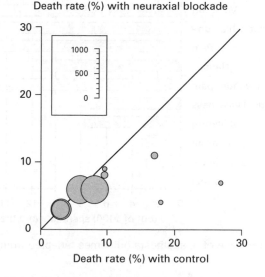

Figure 3.5 Nine trials with at least 10 deaths per trial

adequate now. For instance, trials of analgesics in acute pain have traditionally been conducted over four to eight hours, because that covered the duration of analgesia for most analgesics. Now, with some analgesics like rofecoxib[7] having longer duration, longer trials have to be done. A systematic review is an opportunity to ask questions about how we do studies, what we measure in studies, why we do studies, and what studies to do.

Size

Most clinical trials are too small, and this is especially the case in anaesthesia and analgesia. Acute postoperative pain studies are often done for regulatory purposes, where the issue is whether a new drug is an analgesic, rather than how effective an analgesic it is. While there is an important place for this sort of study, to be clinically relevant studies have to be much larger than the traditional 40 patients per group, perhaps 10 times larger. This is also a problem with studies of postoperative nausea and vomiting (PONV), where similar patients having similar interventions can have PONV rates that vary between 0% and 100%, in part because they are tiny. No such trial can be of any value, except as a marketing exercise, which so many are.

Outcomes

Systematic reviews can help us focus on what we measure in clinical trials. It is easy to measure that which is measurable, but we have to

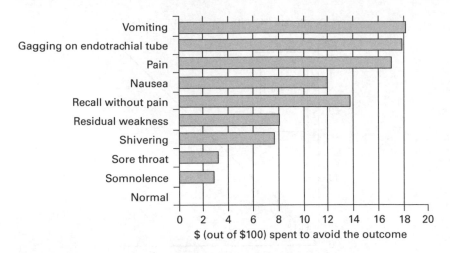

Figure 3.6 Relative value of anaesthesia outcomes. Adapted from[8] with permission

think more about what is important. This can mean important to patients, or professionals, or institutions. Knowing what is important to patients is rare, but for anaesthesia we have at least one study that gives some insight.[8]

This Stanford study began with a literature search for anaesthetic outcomes and complications to generate a comprehensive list of clinical anaesthetic outcomes. Simple descriptions of each outcome were then developed for each. The relative value of 10 items was evaluated. Patients were asked to rank order the 10 possible postoperative outcomes, with 1 being the most undesirable and 10 the most desirable. They were then asked in the relative value section to distribute an imaginary $100 on their preferences such that the more money they spent on it, the *less* likely it was to occur.

A random number generator was used to select a target 100 patients, over the age of 18, who were scheduled for surgery either in an outpatient centre or a main hospital suite. Before the operation, patients ranked vomiting, gagging, pain, and nausea as the worst outcomes. They also gave these four outcomes a high relative value (Figure 3.6). A normal outcome was ranked the most useful outcome, and none of the $100 was spent to avoid it.

Why we do studies

Doing a systematic review is a humbling business. The first thing it teaches is just how much poor-quality work has been done, or work with little or no relevance. It is not uncommon to exclude because of obvious flaws between one and 10 papers for every one that is included. And then, in a second round, as the included papers are read in detail, even more are excluded for less obvious reasons, which could be something as simple as not mentioning how many patients were studied. And then again, one finds that studies have obvious mistakes in calculation or in statistics,[9] perhaps as many as one in 10. Doing a systematic review before starting new clinical research helps individuals and groups determine their objectives.

What studies to do

A criticism of anaesthesia and analgesia could be that many studies are done for neither academic nor pragmatic reasons, but to provide a boost to curricula vitae or as a marketing exercise for companies. A small randomised trial is relatively easy to do, and one review of propofol included well over 100 randomised trials, most of which were small.[10] Is this good enough?

The fact is that, in many cases, we have effective treatments but do not use them effectively. Postoperative analgesia should be straightforward given the number of effective measures at our disposal, from spinal opiates and patient-controlled intravenous opiates to oral non-steroidal anti-inflammatory drugs and now cyclooxygenase inhibitors (COXIBs) of long duration. Yet, surveys continue to show that a large number of patients in hospital experience moderate or severe pain, and even general practitioners have problems with patients sent home after ambulatory surgery.[11]

So, our systematic review of interventions for acute pain may help us decide to do a different sort of trial. Not, perhaps, yet another small randomised trial of treatment A versus treatment B, but rather a study of the clinical effects of re-engineering the processes involved with the delivery of postoperative analgesia.

Conclusion

There are, therefore, a number of reasons why we need systematic reviews in anaesthesia and analgesia. Systematic reviews are essential research tools for clinical research that can, and often should, have relevance for clinical practice. That is not to be confused with any arguments about the place of evidence-based medicine in a complex and often confusing world, though systematic reviews will be a cornerstone of evidence-based medicine too. There are places where systematic reviews will be a waste of time, like diagnostic testing, where almost all trials have structures that are so biased that it makes a systematic review a waste of time, and almost certainly misleading.

Systematic reviews are simple research tools. If done well, they can inform. Doing them, or reading one, should always make us think. They demand that we do better, and better thoughtout, research in the future.

References

1. Counsell CE, Clarke MJ, Slattery J, Sandercock PAG. The miracle of DICE therapy for acute stroke: fact or fictional product of subgroup analysis? *BMJ* 1994;**309**:1677–81.
2. Moore RA, Gavaghan D, Tramèr MR, Collins SL, McQuay, HJ. Size is everything – large amounts of information are needed to overcome random effects in estimating direction and magnitude of treatment effects. *Pain* 1998;**78**:209–16.
3. Naylor CD, Chen E, Strauss B. Measured enthusiasm: does the method of reporting trial results alter perceptions of therapeutic effectiveness? *Ann Intern Med* 1992;**117**:916–21.
4. Rodgers A, Walker N, Schug S, *et al*. Reduction in postoperative mortality and morbidity with epidural or spinal anaesthesia: results from overview of randomised trials. *BMJ* 2000;**321**:1–12.
5. Rigg JR, Jamrozik K, Myles PS, *et al*. MASTER Anaethesia Trial Study Group. Epidural anaesthesia and analgesia and outcome of major surgery: a randomised trial. *Lancet* 2002;**359**:1276–82.
6. Park WY, Thompson JS, Lee, KK. Effect of epidural anesthesia and analgesia on perioperative outcome: a randomized, controlled Veteran Affairs cooperative study. *Ann Surg* 2001;**234**:560–9.
7. Barden J, Edwards JE, McQuay HJ, Moore RA. Single-dose rofecoxib for acute postoperative pain in adults: a quantitative systematic review. *BMC Anesthesiology* 2002;**2**:4. www.biomedcentral.com/1471-2253/2/4 (accessed 21 March 2003).
8. Macario A, Weinger M, Carney S, Kim A. Which clinical anesthesia outcomes are important to avoid? The perspective of patients. *Anesth Analg* 1999;**89**:652–8.
9. Smith LA, Oldman AD, McQuay HJ, Moore RA. Teasing apart quality and validity in systematic reviews: an example from acupuncture trials in chronic neck and back pain. *Pain* 2000;**86**:119–32.
10. Tramèr M, Moore A, McQuay H. Propofol and bradycardia: causation, frequency and severity. *Br J Anaesth* 1997;**78**:642–51.
11. Robaux S, Bouaziz H, Cornet C, Boivin JM, Lefèvre N, Laxenaire MC. Acute postoperative pain management at home after ambulatory surgery: a French pilot survey of general practitioners' views. *Anesth Analg* 2002;**95**:1258–62.

Part II
Systematic reviews in anaesthesia and analgesia

Part II

4: Acute pain

HENRY J MCQUAY

Perhaps the traditional way to write a chapter on acute pain is to begin by lamenting the current state of affairs, and then to go on to discuss the latest fashionable intervention. Acute pain is no different from other areas of medicine, in that we all have strong opinions, and often the stronger the opinion the weaker is the underlying evidence. This chapter will have a short lament and then will summarise efforts to gather evidence for simple interventions. Wherever possible, recommendations are based on systematic reviews of randomised trials, because these provide the highest level of evidence of the efficacy of our interventions. We are fortunate that there is now a steady supply of systematic reviews in the pain world.[1] Obviously, the good evidence now available from systematic reviews about the relative efficacy of oral analgesics in moderate and severe postoperative pain should improve postoperative care. More general clinical recommendations have been covered elsewhere.[2]

There are aspects of collecting evidence in acute pain which, however, receive much less attention than the collection of the efficacy evidence. One of these is the risk of harm. We are much less clear about the rules for collecting evidence about harm than we are about the rules for efficacy. We are all learning that if we want credible estimates of efficacy then these need to be taken from trials that are themselves credible and valid. The simplest starting point to assure such credibility and validity is that for efficacy we should look only to trials that are randomised to control for selection bias and double-blind to control for observer bias. If we stray from this quality standard then we are likely to overestimate treatment efficacy substantially.[3] With common adverse effects, reasonable estimates of incidence may be detected in randomised trials. Rare (serious) adverse effects are not likely to be detected in small randomised trials, and evidence from study architectures that are technically weaker than randomised trials may not only be admissible but crucial. As a simple example, if we have not seen a serious adverse effect in 1500 patients exposed to the treatment – the average number "exposed" when a drug is registered – then we can be 95% confident that the worst possible incidence of a serious adverse effect is 3 divided by 1500, or 1 in 500 patients.[4] If you decided that 1 in 5000 was an acceptable level of risk of a serious adverse effect, then you would have to study 15 000 patients and not see such a problem to be 95% confident that the risk was indeed 1 in 5000.

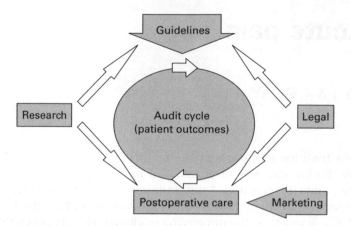

Figure 4.1 Influences on postoperative care

A second problem area is the implementation of the ideas that flow from the collection of evidence. There is a complicated relationship between evidence, guidelines, research, and legal considerations, and the patients' outcomes as assessed by audit (Figure 4.1). Guidelines can only be as good as the evidence that goes into them. If the evidence is thin, then we need to know that.

A minor lament

Of course, pain should be well controlled. Patients should not have to stay unduly long in hospital because of poor pain relief; neither should they have to contact healthcare professionals for pain relief after they have left hospital. High-quality postoperative care needs effective pain management. Although we would like to believe that we practice good pain control, a survey of 5150 recently discharged patients from 36 UK hospitals showed that, for the 3163 who responded to questions on pain, practice was far from ideal[5] (Table 4.1).

It is hard to be precise about the effect that poorly controlled pain has on the incidence of patients having to stay in hospital, or on the incidence of consultations after leaving hospital. After day surgery, ideal targets seem to be that less than 1% should have to stay, and less than 1% should have to consult.[6] Audits have shown that poor pain control can certainly produce higher rates than 1% for both categories,[7] and that providing better pain control produced a worthwhile reduction in both types of problem.

Beyond the humanitarian motive of delivering effective pain control, there is the issue of whether or not good pain control speeds recovery. There is still no compelling evidence that this is so. We may be able to show that a particular technique has an advantage over others on one

Table 4.1 Inpatient survey		
Question answered	**No of patients**	**Percentage**
Pain was present all or most of the time	1042/3162	33
Pain was severe or moderate	2755/3157	87
Pain was worse than expected	182/1051	17
Had to ask for drugs	1085/2589	42
Drugs did not arrive immediately	455/1085	42

Adapted from[5]

aspect of recovery – for instance, the use of epidural analgesia for reducing postoperative pulmonary morbidity[8] – but this is not the same as showing that we are speeding up recovery. Evidence that good pain management led to faster recovery would increase the pressure to improve current practice, which (lamentably) is often less than ideal.

For the final verse for the lament, it would be naïve to assume that postoperative care is "just" a collection of interventions. It is a package of care that needs to be examined as a whole, as well as in its parts. Publications that analyse the process of postoperative care provision are rare, just as they are in other areas of medicine, perhaps because they attract few academic plaudits. There is good evidence that the risk of adverse events is increased when high-tech approaches are used for drug administration,[9] so that implementing high-tech packages because low-tech is working poorly should not be done without thinking about the risks. Perhaps the low-tech package could be better delivered, by improving its efficacy and maintaining lower levels of risk.

Amassing useful evidence

For acute pain we are not interested in treatments that do not work. The question is not does the treatment work?, but rather, how well does it work? Perhaps, surprisingly, there are few credible comparisons of one technique with another. One reason is simply history – we have inherited several drugs with time-honoured efficacy in acute pain, and the necessary time, money, and energy to compare all the various contenders head-to-head has not been forthcoming.

Although we do not have a plentiful supply of randomised trials comparing treatment x with treatment y, we do have randomised trials that compare the different drugs with placebo. An analogy here is with a 100 m track. We can ask people to race against each other on the track – the head-to-head comparison. Alternatively, we can ask them to run against the clock, rather than against each other. This would give us a listing of times from which we can produce a ranking, from fastest through to slowest. For this to be fair we need to ensure that the conditions were the same for each competitor and that we had the same timing method. Given such caveats, we would have useful information about who was the quickest and who was the slowest, even if we could not manage to have them all race head-to-head against each other.

We have used the run-against-the-clock method to develop league tables, or rank orderings, for which analgesic works best after surgery. We have done this because we have developed ways of using the randomised trials that compare the different drugs with placebo so that we can compare their relative performance. This has involved developing new methods and extending existing ones, which are documented elsewhere.[10,11] Although the information we all want is the league table, the credibility of that league table rests on the credibility of the methods used to compile it. The intention is to provide clinically useful information. In an ideal world one would have head-to-head comparisons of all the interventions in which one was interested. In reality these do not exist. Although the relative ranking method is theoretically inferior, because the comparisons are not made within the same randomisation so that conditions might not have been the same for each competitor, we would contend that the utility of the relative ranking far outweighs the theoretical (and acknowledged) disadvantage. We have to treat now to the best of our ability, not wait until something better comes along – which, of course, might never happen.

For the work reported here, we obtained all the trials of a particular drug compared with placebo in postoperative pain. The drug's performance in the trials was then converted into a common currency: the proportion of patients with moderate or severe postoperative pain who achieve at least 50% pain relief compared with placebo over six hours.

Non-opioids: paracetamol, combinations, and non-steroidal anti-inflammatory drugs

Effective relief can be achieved with oral non-opioids and non-steroidal anti-inflammatory drugs (NSAIDs). These drugs are appropriate for many post-surgical and post-traumatic pains, especially when patients go home on the day of their operation. Figure 4.2 shows the evolving league table for analgesic efficacy compiled from randomised trials after all kinds of surgery. Analgesic efficacy is expressed as the number needed to treat (NNT) – the number of patients who need to receive the active drug for one to achieve at least 50% relief of pain compared with placebo over a six-hour treatment period. The most effective drugs have a low NNT of just over 2, meaning that for every two patients who receive the drug, one patient will get at least 50% relief because of the treatment (the other patient may obtain relief but it does not reach the 50% level). For

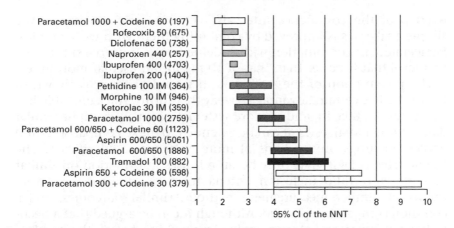

Figure 4.2 League table of relative efficacy for some common analgesics. Number needed to treat (NNT; number in parenthesis is total in comparison) for at least 50% pain relief over 4–6 hours in patients with moderate-to-severe pain. All are oral analgesics except intramuscular (IM) morphine, pethidine, and ketorolac

paracetamol 1 g, the NNT is about 4. The combination of paracetamol 1 g with codeine 60 mg improves the NNT to just over 2.

The NNT is treatment specific, and is drug, dose, and context specific. In these special circumstances NNT is useful for comparing relative efficacy. Because the NNT comparisons here are against placebo, the best NNT of 2 means that 50 of 100 patients, who would not have gained relief with placebo, will get at least 50% relief specifically because of the treatment. Another 10–20 will have had adequate pain relief with placebo, giving them at least 50% relief. With ibuprofen 400 mg, therefore, about 60 of 100 patients in total will have effective pain relief. For comparison, with 10 mg intramuscular morphine about 50% of patients receive more than 50% pain relief. Because the effect of placebo is added in when looking at percentages with an outcome of at least 50% pain relief, the comparisons between analgesics are not as stark as with NNT.

Figure 4.2 shows information on oral paracetamol, paracetamol plus codeine, and several NSAIDs from systematic reviews of randomised controlled trials of single doses in postoperative pain. It is clear that the oral NSAIDs do extremely well in this single-dose postoperative comparison. They all have NNT values of between 2 and 3, and the point estimate of the mean is below that of (that is, better than) 10 mg of intramuscular morphine, even though the confidence intervals overlap. The simple analgesics, aspirin and paracetamol, are significantly less effective than 10 mg intramuscular morphine. The point estimates of the NNT are higher, and there is no overlap of the confidence intervals. The analgesic efficacy of the simple analgesics is improved by combining them with weak opioids. Paracetamol in combination with codeine lowers (improves) the NNT to a level that is better than that of 10 mg intramuscular morphine.

The presentation of the NNT data in graphical form as shown in Figure 4.2 has certain advantages over other forms. A league table like this is easy to take in, and as more systematic reviews compile similar data on other analgesics, it can be extended to make comparisons and choices of drugs on the basis of more evidence-based efficacy. The league table is legitimate only because it uses information on similar patients with valid inclusion criteria (pain of moderate or severe intensity), similar measurement methods, similar outcomes, and a common comparator, placebo. Although it can be argued that a head-to-head comparison between analgesics would be better, the problem is that few such head-to-head comparisons exist, and randomised trials to detect small differences in efficacy between two analgesics would need to be massive to be able to detect differences in direction, let alone in the magnitude of the difference.[12]

The clear message is that, of the oral analgesics, NSAIDs perform the best, and that paracetamol alone or in combination with other drugs is also effective. The strongest oral analgesic regimen would be an oral NSAID supplemented as necessary with paracetamol and opioid. As the pain wanes, the prescription should become paracetamol based, supplemented if necessary by an NSAID. When used in day surgery, a regimen like this resulted in high-quality pain relief without recourse to general practitioner visits.[7]

Injected analgesics – opioids and NSAIDs

Using the same methods, we have obtained information on intramuscular pethidine and ketorolac.[13] If this information is considered together with the intramuscular morphine data shown above, we can then start to think about the optimal choice within and between drug class for intramuscular injection, and indeed about the optimal choice of route of administration.

We sought, as for the oral drugs in the league table (Figure 4.2), published randomised controlled trials in which single doses, injected or oral, of pethidine and ketorolac were compared with placebo in moderate-to-severe postoperative pain. Information about summed pain intensity or pain relief outcomes over four to six hours was extracted, and converted into dichotomous information, for the number of patients with at least 50% pain relief. This was then used to calculate the relative risk and the NNT for one patient to achieve at least 50% pain relief. Minor and major adverse effect data were extracted and summarised.

Table 4.2. Regional analgesia summary

		Indications	Advantages	Problems
Low-tech	Topical wound infiltration	Surface surgery	Simple	Short duration
		Most wounds	Simple	Short duration
	Peripheral nerve blocks	Limb surgery/ trauma	Catheter possible	Nerve damage
			Catheter possible	Motor block
	Plexus blocks	Limb surgery		
High-tech	Epidural (including caudal)	Major surgery (thoraco–abdominal, lower limb)	Catheter possible Reduced thrombo-embolism	Adverse effects surveillance
	Intrathecal	Major surgery (thoraco-abdominal, lower limb)	Long-duration relief possible from single injection of low-dose opioid	Adverse effects surveillance

For pethidine, eight randomised controlled trials of intramuscular (IM) doses met our inclusion criteria, with 254 patients having been given pethidine and 214 given placebo. A single 100 mg dose of intramuscular pethidine, but not pethidine 50 mg, significantly benefited patients, compared with placebo (Figure 4.2). The NNT for at least 50% pain relief was 2·9 (95% confidence interval 2·3–3·9). Pethidine 100 mg IM produced significantly more drowsiness or somnolence and dizziness or light-headedness than placebo, with numbers-needed-to-harm (NNH) of 2·9 (2·2–4·4) and 7·2 (4·8–14), respectively.

Fourteen reports met the inclusion criteria for ketorolac, six for IM and eight for oral drug administration. A dose–response was available for IM ketorolac. Most information was available for the 30 mg dose, which had a NNT of 3·4 (2·5–4·9). There was also a dose–response for oral ketorolac. Most information was available for the 10 mg dose, which had a NNT of 2·6 (2·3–3·1). Over the dose ranges studied, oral ketorolac was consistently about three times more potent than IM ketorolac. Only with oral ketorolac 10 mg were any adverse events statistically more frequent than with placebo, with a relative risk of 7.3 (4.7–17).

The intramuscular analgesic efficacy of pethidine 100 mg was comparable to ketorolac 30 mg when given as a single postoperative dose for moderate-to-severe pain and similar to IM morphine 10 mg. Oral ketorolac 10 mg produced similar efficacy. The adverse effects for IM pethidine 100 mg were similar in type and frequency to those found with morphine 10 mg. By contrast, adverse effects with ketorolac 30 mg IM were not significantly more common than with placebo.

Pulling all this efficacy evidence together

Some selected results from the league tables for oral and intramuscular analgesics are shown in Figure 4.2. It is clear that oral NSAIDs perform as well as morphine 10 mg or pethidine 100 mg. Also, there is little difference in the efficacy of oral and injected ketorolac. These two facts may seem counterintuitive, but in reality they have been known for many years from head-to-head comparisons of oral NSAID and injected opioid, and of injected versus oral NSAID. Examples are:

- injecting morphine at a dose of 10 mg provides similar analgesia to oral NSAID[14]
- injecting morphine at doses of 10–20 mg provides similar analgesia to injected NSAID[15]
- injecting NSAID provides similar analgesia to oral NSAID[16,17]
- injecting 20 mg of morphine provides greater analgesia than injecting 10 mg, and greater analgesia than the best performers on the oral league table.[15]

Perhaps the results simply seem more obvious when plotted like this. In particular, the comparison is very useful when addressing some of the following:

- if patients can swallow, the oral route should be preferred
- which classes of drugs are the most effective postoperative analgesics (or which are least effective)?
- how well do injections perform compared with the oral drugs? Within a class of drugs does the same dose work better when injected than when taken orally?
- when should we consider using techniques such as epidurals or spinals?
- when should we supplement with injections of local anaesthetic?
- should we be using prophylaxis or treating-as-necessary – are the arguments for prophylaxis convincing?

Even if patients can swallow, is it best to give drugs by injection or suppository?

Most postoperative pain is managed solely with medication. Perhaps because anaesthetists work with injected drugs there is a natural belief that drugs that are injected are more powerful than drugs taken by mouth.

It is important to know which oral analgesics to recommend to patients because so much postoperative care now takes place in the home. We are biased to think of patients after major surgery, but they too need oral analgesics when they can swallow.

There is an old adage that if patients can swallow, it is best to take drugs by mouth. There is no evidence that NSAIDs given rectally or by injection perform better than the same drug at the same dose given by mouth;[13,18] two randomised, double-blind, placebo-controlled comparisons failed to distinguish any difference between oral ibuprofen arginine 400 mg and intramuscular ketorolac 30 mg.[16,17] These other non-oral routes become appropriate when patients cannot swallow. Topical NSAIDs are effective in acute musculoskeletal injuries – ibuprofen has a NNT of 3 for at least 50% relief at one week compared with placebo.[19]

The patient can't swallow analgesics

The emerging information on the relative efficacy of injected opioids or NSAIDs indicates (Figure 4.2) that there is probably little difference in efficacy between say morphine 10 mg and ketorolac 30 mg. The non-opioid advantage of the NSAID may, however, be ruled out if there is concern over adverse effects. Adverse-effect data on NSAIDs from long-term oral dosing, where gastric bleeding is the main worry, rate ibuprofen as the safest.[20] The main concerns in acute pain are renal and coagulation problems. Acute renal failure can be precipitated in patients with pre-existing heart or kidney disease, those on loop diuretics, or those who have lost more than 10% of blood volume. NSAIDs cause significant lengthening (~30%) of bleeding time, but usually still within the normal range. This can last for days with aspirin or hours with non-aspirin NSAIDs. Whether or not NSAIDs cause significant increase in blood loss remains contentious.[21] Importantly, increasing the dose of opioid will increase analgesia. Injecting 20 mg of morphine gave greater analgesia than 10 mg.[22] Increasing the dose of NSAID may not produce as steep an increase in the analgesic effect as occurs with opioids.

Other drugs

As yet, we do not have any systematic review evidence for several "niche" analgesic interventions. These include inhaled nitrous oxide, which can provide fast-onset–fast-offset analgesia for obstetrics and wound dressings, corticosteroids to reduce pain and swelling after head and neck surgery and when swelling causes pain in cancer, ketamine in emergency analgesia and anaesthesia, and clonidine.

Opioids

For severe acute pain, opioids are the first-line treatment and, to date, we have few systematic reviews – for injected morphine[22] and for injected pethidine.[13] Intermittent opioid injection can provide effective relief of acute pain.[23] Unfortunately, adequate doses are withheld because of traditions, misconceptions, ignorance, and fear. Doctors and nurses fear addiction and respiratory depression. Addiction is not a problem with opioid use in acute pain. Over 11 000 patients were followed up a year after opioids were given for acute pain, and just four were considered to be addicts.[24]

Irrespective of the route of administration, opioids used for people who are not in pain, or in doses larger than necessary to control the pain, can slow or indeed stop breathing. The key principle is to titrate the dose against the desired effect – pain relief – and minimise unwanted effects (Figure 4.3). If the patient is still complaining of pain and you are sure that the drug has all been delivered and absorbed, then it is safe to give another, usually smaller, dose (5 min after intravenous, 1 hour after intramuscular or subcutaneous, 90 min after oral). If the second dose is also ineffective, then repeat the process or change the route of administration to achieve faster control. Delayed-release formulations, oral or transdermal, should not be used in acute pain because delayed onset and offset are dangerous in this context.

There is no compelling evidence that one opioid is better than another, but there is good evidence that pethidine has a specific disadvantage[25] and no specific advantage. Given in multiple doses, the metabolite norpethidine can accumulate and act as a central nervous system irritant, ultimately causing convulsions, especially in renal dysfunction. Pethidine should not be used when multiple injections are needed. The old idea that pethidine is better than other opioids at dealing with colicky pain is no longer tenable.[26]

Morphine (and its relatives diamorphine and codeine) has an active rather than a toxic metabolite, morphine-6-glucuronide. In renal dysfunction this metabolite can accumulate and result in greater effect from a given dose because it is more active than morphine. If you are, as you should be, titrating dose against effect, this will not matter. Less morphine will be needed. Accumulation can be a problem with unconscious intensive care patients on fixed dose schedules when renal function is compromised.

Opioid-induced adverse effects include nausea and vomiting, constipation, sedation, pruritus, urinary retention, and respiratory depression. There is no good evidence that the incidence is different with different opioids at the same level of analgesia. There is good evidence that the risk of adverse events is increased when high-tech approaches are used for drug administration.[9]

There are strong arguments, based on minimising risk, for using one opioid only, so that everyone involved is familiar with dosage, effects, and problems. Our first choice opioid is morphine. Whichever drug you choose, simple changes to the way opioids are used, good staff

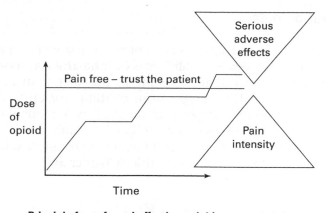

Principle for safe and effective opioid use –
titrate to effect

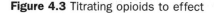

If the patient is asking for more opioid it
usually signals inadequate pain control:

Too little drug
Too long between doses
Too little attention paid to the patient
Too much reliance on rigid (inadequate) prescriptions

Figure 4.3 Titrating opioids to effect

education, and implementation of an algorithm for intermittent
opioid dosing can have a powerful impact on pain relief and patient
satisfaction.[23]

Intermittent opioid injection by nurses requires good staffing levels
to minimise delay between need and injection. Staffing shortage,
ward distractions, and controlled drug regulations all increase the
delay. Patient-controlled analgesia overcomes these logistical
problems. The patient presses a button and receives a pre-set dose of
opioid from a syringe driver connected to an intravenous or
subcutaneous cannula. This delivers opioid to the same opioid
receptors as an intermittent injection, but allows the patient to
circumvent delays. Not surprisingly, there is little difference in
outcome between efficient intermittent injection and patient-
controlled analgesia.[27,28] Good risk management with patient-
controlled analgesia should emphasise the same drug, protocols, and
equipment throughout the hospital.

Novel routes of opioid administration, intended to improve
analgesia and reduce adverse effects, include intra-articular,[29] nasal,
active transdermal, and inhalational. These may prove to have an
advantage over conventional routes, different kinetic profiles, or
greater convenience, but their place in mainstream care is unproven.

Peripheral opioids

At least for intra-articular peripheral opioids, the story becomes a little clearer. A systematic review of valid trials of intra-articular morphine in knee surgery has shown that morphine in the knee joint can indeed provide analgesia.[29,30] This analgesia can continue for up to 24 hours, although there is no dose–response available. It is the long duration of action that suggests this technique might have practical application beyond its research interest.[31] For peripheral opioids injected into other sites, the evidence for efficacy is very thin (Chapter 5).[32]

Regional analgesia

The technical advantage of regional analgesia with local anaesthetic is that it can deliver complete pain relief by interrupting pain transmission from a localised area, so avoiding generalised drug adverse effects. This advantage is more obvious when further doses can be given via a catheter, extending the duration of analgesia. Details are given in Table 4.2.

There is a necessary distinction between anaesthetic blocks done to permit surgery, and blocks done together with a general anaesthetic to provide postoperative pain relief. There is clear evidence that blocks can indeed provide good relief in the initial postoperative period,[33] and no evidence to suggest that patients with blocks then experience "rebound", and need more postoperative pain relief. The risk of neurological damage is the major drawback,[34] and ideally blocks should not be done on anaesthetised patients.

Epidural analgesia

Epidural infusion via a catheter can offer continuous relief after trauma or surgery, for lower limb, spine, abdominal region, or chest. The current optimal infusate is an opioid–local anaesthetic mixture. Opioids and local anaesthetics have a synergistic effect, so that lower doses of each are required for equivalent analgesia with fewer adverse effects.[35]

The risks are those of an epidural (dural puncture, infection, haematoma, nerve damage), the local anaesthetic (hypotension, motor block, toxicity), and the opioid, (nausea, sedation, urinary retention, respiratory depression, pruritus) (Box 4.1). Wrong doses do get given,[9] so increased surveillance is mandatory. The risk of persistent neurological sequelae after an epidural is about 1 in 5000.[36] Debate continues about whether patients with epidural infusions can be nursed on general wards. These techniques are only appropriate for major trauma or surgery when the potential benefits outweigh the risks.

Box 4.1 Adverse effects of regional analgesia

- Needle or catheter damage to nerves, pleura, dura, or viscus
- Intravenous injection of local anaesthetic
- Overdose of local anaesthetic
- Motor block
- Autonomic blockade – hypotension, urinary retention
- Respiratory depression (spinal opioids)

Why epidurals are important in acute pain

Asking radical questions about acute postoperative management, such as, why are all operations not ambulatory, pain-free, and risk-free? or, more familiar, why is this patient still in hospital?, is forcing a reconsideration of the role of combined (local or regional plus general anaesthesia) approaches. Instead of asking questions such as is regional better than general anaesthesia? we need to look at the whole episode, before, during, and after surgery, not just at the operative period (Chapter 14).[37,38] Costs of each care episode should fall if the hospital stay is reduced, and a healthy patient returned home will cost the community less than a sick patient requiring considerable input from the primary care team. Our old question was whether regional or regional-supplemented general anaesthesia could produce major reductions in morbidity and mortality – the general versus regional anaesthesia question. An example is vascular surgery. The Yeager study[39] did suggest improvement with regional anaesthesia in patients undergoing abdominal aortic aneurysm or lower extremity vascular surgery. A feature of subsequent studies that showed no difference between regional and general anaesthesia was an increasing extent of control over all aspects of postoperative care.[40,41] The effect of the detailed protocols was that bad outcomes were reduced in all groups.[42] The implication is that even if there was a difference it would take a huge study to show it using the morbidity and mortality outcomes.[43] But the suggestion is that it is only if the postoperative protocols allow any advantage to be expressed, such as advantage in time to feeding or time to walking, that we will see a difference between regional and general anaesthesia. Epidural local anaesthetic may well allow bowel function to return earlier,[44] but only if protocol allows it will we see patients going home two days after major surgery.[45] The point is that this radical change is only possible if the procedure is done under an epidural, because the epidural makes it possible for the patient to mobilise early and for bowel function to return earlier.

For some operations there is proven advantage of regional anaesthesia over general anaesthesia. For hip[46] and knee[47] replacements "solid" epidural anaesthesia with sedation during surgery followed by postoperative epidural can reduce blood loss, produce faster surgery, reduce morbidity, and produce faster rehabilitation. In this context, change has been gradual rather than radical, but again the key is the epidural, both for the operation and afterwards.

Returning to the old question – general versus regional anaesthesia – a recent set of meta-analyses looked at randomised controlled trials to assess the effects of seven different interventions on postoperative pulmonary function after a variety of procedures.[8] The seven were epidural opioid, epidural local anaesthetic, epidural opioid with local anaesthetic, thoracic versus lumbar epidural opioid, intercostal nerve block, wound infiltration with local anaesthetic, and intrapleural local anaesthetic. Compared with systemic opioids, epidural opioids decreased the incidence of atelectasis significantly. Epidural local anaesthetics compared with systemic opioids increased PaO_2 significantly and decreased the incidence of pulmonary infections and pulmonary complications overall. Intercostal nerve blockade did not produce significant improvement in pulmonary outcome measures.

Other techniques

With specialised procedures, such as paravertebral or interpleural injections, we seldom have head-to-head comparisons with standard treatment. This is frustrating, because in highly skilled hands these procedures appear to perform well. What we have is can-do evidence, but what we need is should-do evidence.

Pain that persists: prophylaxis or wait until it happens?

One of the intriguing problems in acute pain is why some patients end up with chronic pain after surgery when others do not. The potential link is between poorly controlled "acute" postoperative pain and perseverance of this pain into a chronic status. A simplistic explanation is that those with chronic pain have nerve damage at surgery. An alternative explanation is that it is the patients with severe postoperative pain who develop the chronic pain. The proposal then follows that if the acute pain was better controlled, the chronic pain would not develop.[48,49] An alternative explanation is that in a proportion of surgical procedures, long-lasting pain will result. This is nothing to do with poor acute pain treatment and nothing to do with the personality of the patient – some people will get long-lasting pain.[50]

Pre-emptive analgesia

The evidence for clinical advantage of giving an intervention before pain as opposed to giving the same intervention after pain is still

(a)

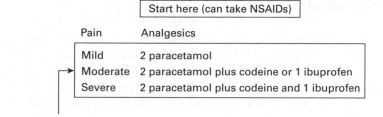

Start here (can take NSAIDs)

Pain	Analgesics
Mild	2 paracetamol
Moderate	2 paracetamol plus codeine or 1 ibuprofen
Severe	2 paracetamol plus codeine and 1 ibuprofen

Wait at least 2 hours
before repeating
cycle

Pain	Analgesics
Mild	none
Moderate	1 ibuprofen
Severe	1 ibuprofen

(b)

Start here (can't take NSAIDs)

Pain	Analgesics
Mild	2 paracetamol
Moderate	1 paracetamol plus codeine and 1 paracetamol
Severe	2 paracetamol plus codeine

Wait at least 4 hours
before repeating
cycle

Pain	Analgesics
Mild	2 paracetamol
Moderate	1 paracetamol plus codeine and 1 paracetamol
Severe	2 paracetamol plus codeine

Figure 4.4 A simple scheme ("three-pot") for acute and chronic pain relief which uses paracetamol alone, paracetamol/opioid combination drugs (a) with and (b) without NSAIDs

unconvincing.[51,52] Certainly, by far the majority of trials of pre-pain versus post-pain dosing have failed to show any clinically meaningful benefit.

TENS and acupuncture

Transcutaneous electrical nerve stimulation (TENS) is not effective for postoperative pain,[53,54] and is of limited value for labour pain.[55]

Systematic reviews of acupuncture in acute pain are problematic, largely because of the poor quality of the trials that are covered in the reviews.[56]

Psychological methods

There is evidence that psychological approaches are beneficial in acute pain.[57] Cognitive behavioural methods can reduce pain and distress in burned patients. Preparation before surgery can reduce postoperative analgesic consumption. The evidence for the use of relaxation and music on postoperative pain is confounded by the poor quality of trials.[58]

Conclusions

The evidence amassed by systematic reviews to date does not answer all the management questions in acute pain, but systematic reviews do provide some of the building blocks necessary for rational decisions. Simple and important is the decision about which oral analgesics to recommend, and especially so after ambulatory surgery.

From the league table (Figure 4.2), two guidelines may be proposed – one for those who can take NSAIDs, one for those who cannot. Basically, there are three analgesics in each of the two guidelines, paracetamol, paracetamol 500 mg plus codeine 30 mg (but other equivalent paracetamol plus opioid combinations would substitute), and an NSAID (ibuprofen 400 mg in this example). Both guidelines minimise exposure to opioid and to NSAID. The schemes are shown in Figure 4.4. This "three-pot" or three-component system is based on best evidence and uses cheapest available analgesics. A similar scheme was used for the Cardiff audit.[7]

References

1. Jadad AR, McQuay HJ. Meta-analyses to evaluate analgesic interventions: a systematic qualitative review of their methodology. *J Clin Epidemiol* 1996;**49**:235–43.
2. McQuay HJ, Justins D, Moore RA. Treating acute pain in hospital. *BMJ* 1997;**314**:1531–5.
3. Schulz KF, Chalmers I, Hayes RJ, Altman DG. Empirical evidence of bias: dimensions of methodological quality associated with estimates of treatment effects in controlled trials. *JAMA* 1995;**273**:408–12.
4. Eypasch E, Lefering R, Kum CK, Troidl H. Probability of adverse events that have not yet occurred: a statistical reminder. *BMJ* 1995;**311**:619–20.
5. Bruster S, Jarman B, Bosanquet N, Weston D, Erens R, Delbanco TL. National survey of hospital patients. *BMJ* 1994;**309**:1542–6.
6. Millar JM, Rudkin GE, Hitchcock M. *Practical anaesthesia and analgesia for day surgery.* Oxford: Bios, 1997.
7. Haynes TK, Evans DEN, Roberts D. Pain relief after day surgery: quality improvement by audit. *J One-day Surg* 1995;**Summer**:12–5.
8. Ballantyne JC, Carr DB, deFerranti S, *et al.* The comparative effects of postoperative analgesic therapies on pulmonary outcome: cumulative meta-analyses of randomized, controlled trials. *Anesth Analg* 1998;**86**:598–612.
9. Bates DW, Cullen DJ, Laird N, *et al.* Incidence of adverse drug events and potential adverse drug events. *JAMA* 1995;**274**:29–34.

10. McQuay HJ, Moore RA. *An evidence-based resource for pain relief.* Oxford: Oxford University Press, 1998.
11. Moore RA, Edwards J, Barden J, McQuay HJ. *Bandolier's Little Book of Pain.* Oxford: Oxford University Press, 2003.
12. Moore RA, Gavaghan D, Tramèr MR, Collins SL, McQuay HJ. Size is everything – large amounts of information are needed to overcome random effects in estimating direction and magnitude of treatment effects. *Pain* 1998;**78**:209–16.
13. Smith LA, Carroll D, Edwards JE, Moore RA, McQuay HJ. Single dose ketorolac and pethidine in acute postoperative pain: a systematic review with meta-analysis. *Br J Anaesthesiol* 2000;**84**:48–58.
14. Mansfield M, Firth F, Glynn C, Kinsella J. A comparison of ibuprofen arginine with morphine sulphate for pain relief after orthopaedic surgery. *Eur J Anaesthesiol* 1996;**13**:492–7.
15. Norholt SE, SindetPedersen S, Larsen U, *et al.* Pain control after dental surgery: a double-blind, randomised trial of lornoxicam versus morphine. *Pain* 1996;**67**:335–43.
16. Laveneziana D, Riva A, Bonazzi M, Cipolla M, Migliavacca S. Comparative efficacy of oral ibuprofen arginine and intramuscular ketorolac in patients with postoperative pain. *Clin Drug Invest* 1996;**11**:8–14.
17. Pagnoni B, Vignali M, Colella S, Monopoli R, Tiengo N. Comparative efficacy of oral ibuprofen arginine and intramuscular ketorolac in patients with postcaesarean section pain. *Clin Drug Invest* 1996;**11**:15–21.
18. Tramèr MR, Williams JE, Carroll D, Wiffen PJ, Moore RA, McQuay HJ. Comparing analgesic efficacy of non-steroidal anti-inflammatory drugs given by different routes in acute and chronic pain: a qualitative systematic review. *Acta Anaesthesiol Scand* 1998;**42**:71–9.
19. Moore RA, Tramèr MR, Carroll D, Wiffen PJ, McQuay HJ. Quantitive systematic review of topically-applied non-steroidal anti-inflammatory drugs. *BMJ* 1998;**316**:333–8.
20. Henry D, Lim LL-Y, Rodriguez LAG, *et al.* Variability in risk of gastrointestinal complications with individual non-steroidal anti-inflammatory drugs: results of a collaborative meta-analysis. *BMJ* 1996;**312**:1563–6.
21. Møiniche S, Rømsing J, Dahl JB, Tramèr MR. Nonsteroidal antiinflammatory drugs and the risk of operative site bleeding after tonsillectomy: a quantitative systematic review. *Anesth Analg* 2003;**96**:68–77.
22. McQuay HJ, Carroll D, Moore RA. Injected morphine in postoperative pain: a quantitative systematic review. *J Pain Sympt Manag* 1999;**17**:164–74.
23. Gould TH, Crosby DL, Harmer M, *et al.* Policy for controlling pain after surgery: effect of sequential changes in management. *BMJ* 1992;**305**:1187–93.
24. Porter J, Jick H. Addiction rate in patients treated with narcotics. *NEJM* 1980;**302**:123.
25. Szeto HH, Inturrisi CE, Houde R, Saal S, Cheigh J, Reidenberg M. Accumulation of norperidine, an active metabolite of meperidine, in patients with renal failure or cancer. *Ann Int Med* 1977;**86**:738–41.
26. Nagle CJ, McQuay HJ. Opiate receptors; their role in effect and side-effect. *Curr Anaesth Crit Care* 1990;**1**:247–52.
27. Ballantyne JC, Carr DB, Chalmers TC, Dear KB, Angelillo IF, Mosteller F. Postoperative patient-controlled analgesia: meta-analyses of initial randomized control trials. *J Clin Anesth* 1993;**5**:182–93.
28. Walder B, Schafer M, Henzi I, Tramèr MR. Efficacy and safety of patient-controlled opioid analgesia for acute postoperative pain: a quantitative systematic review. *Acta Anaesthesiol Scand* 2001;**45**:795–804.
29. Kalso E, Tramèr M, Carroll D, McQuay H, Moore RA. Pain relief from intra-articular morphine after knee surgery: a qualitative systematic review. *Pain* 1997;**71**:642–51.
30. Kalso E, Smith L, McQuay HJ, Moore RA. No pain, no gain: clinical excellence and scientific rigour – lessons learned from IA morphine. *Pain* 2002;**98**:269–75.
31. Kanbak NM, Akpolat N, Öcal T, Doral NM, Ercan M, Erdem K. Intraarticular morphine administration provides pain relief after knee arthroscopy. *Eur J Anaesthesiol* 1997;**14**:153–6.
32. Picard PR, Tramèr MR, McQuay HJ, Moore RA. Analgesic efficacy of peripheral opioids (all except intra-articular): a qualitative systematic review of randomised controlled trials. *Pain* 1997;**72**:309–18.

33. McQuay HJ, Carroll D, Moore RA. Postoperative orthopaedic pain: the effect of opiate premedication and local anaesthetic blocks. *Pain* 1988;**33**:291–5.
34. Bridenbaugh PO. Complications of local anesthetic neural blockade. In: Cousins MJ, Bridenbaugh PO, eds. *Neural Blockade*. Philadelphia: Lippincott, 1988;695–717.
35. McQuay HJ, Moore RA. Local anaesthetics and epidurals. In: Wall PD, Melzack R, eds. *Textbook of Pain*. Edinburgh: Churchill Livingstone, 1999;1215–31.
36. Kane RE. Neurologic deficits following epidural or spinal anesthesia. *Anesth Analg* 1981;**60**:150–61.
37. Kehlet H. Multimodal approach to control postoperative pathophysiology and rehabilitation. *Br J Anaesth* 1997;**78**:606–17.
38. Kehlet H. Postoperative pain relief: what is the issue? *Br J Anaesth* 1994;**72**:375–8.
39. Yeager M, Glass D, Neff R, Brinck-Johnsen T. Epidural anaesthesia and analgesia in high risk surgical patients. *Anesthesiology* 1987;**66**:729–36.
40. Bode RJ, Lewis KP, Zarich SW, *et al*. Cardiac outcome after peripheral vascular surgery: comparison of general and regional anesthesia. *Anesthesiology* 1996;**84**:3–13.
41. Christopherson R, Beattie C, Frank SM, *et al*. Perioperative morbidity in patients randomized to epidural or general anesthesia for lower extremity vascular surgery. Perioperative Ischemia Randomized Anesthesia Trial Study Group. *Anesthesiology* 1993;**79**:422–34.
42. Beattie C, Roizen MF, Downing JW. Cardiac outcomes after regional or general anesthesia: do we know the question? *Anesthesiology* 1996;**85**:1207–9.
43. Rigg JRA, Jamrozik K. Outcome after general or regional anaesthesia in high-risk patients. *Curr Opin Anaesthesiol* 1998;**11**:327–31.
44. Liu SS, Carpenter RL, Mackey DC, *et al*. Effects of perioperative analgesic technique on rate of recovery after colon surgery. *Anesthesiology* 1995;**83**:757–65.
45. Bardram L, Funch-Jensen P, Jensen P, Crawford ME, Kehlet H. Recovery after laparoscopic colonic surgery with epidural analgesia, and early oral nutrition and mobilisation. *Lancet* 1995;**345**:763–4.
46. Sharrock NE, Salvati EA. Hypotensive epidural anesthesia for total hip arthroplasty: a review. *Acta Orthopaed Scand* 1996;**67**:91–107.
47. Williams-Russo P, Sharrock NE, Haas SB, *et al*. Randomized trial of epidural versus general anesthesia: outcomes after primary total knee replacement. *Clin Orth Rel Res* 1996;199–208.
48. Eija K, Tiina T, Pertti NJ. Amitriptyline effectively relieves neuropathic pain following treatment of breast cancer. *Pain* 1996;**64**:293–302.
49. Katz J, Jackson M, Kavanagh BP, Sandler A. Acute pain after thoracic surgery predicts long-term post-thoracotomy pain. *Clin J Pain* 1996;**12**:50–5.
50. Perkins FM, Kehlet H. Chronic pain as an outcome of surgery. *Anesthesiology* 2000;**93**:1123–33.
51. McQuay HJ. Pre-emptive analgesia: a systematic review of clinical studies. *Ann Med* 1995;**27**:249–56.
52. Møiniche S, Kehlet H, Dahl JB. A qualitative and quantitative systematic review of preemptive analgesia for postoperative pain relief. *Anesthesiology* 2002;**96**:725–41.
53. Reeve J, Menon D, Corabian P. Transcutaneous electrical nerve stimulation (TENS): a technology assessment. *Int J Technol Ass Health Care* 1996;**12**:299–324.
54. Carroll D, Tramèr M, McQuay H, Nye B, Moore A. Randomization is important in studies with pain outcomes: systematic review of transcutaneous electrical stimulation in acute postoperative pain. *Br J Anaesth* 1996;**77**:798–803.
55. Carroll D, Tramèr M, McQuay H, Nye B, Moore A. Transcutaneous electrical nerve stimulation in labour pain: a systematic review. *Br J Obstet Gynaecol* 1997;**104**:169–75.
56. Ernst E, Pittler MH. The effectiveness of acupuncture in treating acute dental pain: a systematic review. *Br Dent J* 1998;**184**:443–7.
57. Justins DM, Richardson PH. Clinical management of acute pain. *Br Med Bull* 1991;**47**:561–83.
58. Good M. Effect of relaxation and music on postoperative pain: a review. *J Adv Nurs* 1996;**24**:905–14.

5: Peripheral treatment of postoperative pain

STEEN MØINICHE, JØRGEN B DAHL

Introduction

In most cases, postoperative pain inevitably follows surgery. It represents one of the most distressing factors that patients face in the post-surgical setting, it interferes with patients' comfort, and it may have an impact on morbidity and convalescence measures. In order to provide the best possible quality for the treatment of postoperative pain, the clinician should have the current best, valid, and relevant information concerning the various treatment options. However, seeking and keeping up with this knowledge have become increasingly difficult tasks as the amount of medical literature on postoperative pain control is expanding exponentially. In December 2002, a Medline search using the search-terms "postoperative pain" and "postoperative analgesia" revealed a number of articles that was well above 15 000. The volume of published medical information has become almost impossible to overview. Concise summaries of available information on treatment of postoperative pain are therefore becoming increasingly important.

The systematic review of postoperative pain treatment

As described thoroughly elsewhere (Chapter 3), the systematic review is a powerful tool to further our understanding of the efficacy and likelihood for harm of interventions by gathering evidence from *all* relevant trials. It is structured to reduce bias in the collection, appraisal, and interpretation of relevant studies by using transparent methodology.[1,2] The methodology includes a definition of a clear, often narrow, question to be answered, a structured literature search with well defined inclusion and exclusion criteria, a quality assessment of retrieved reports, and standardised data handling and analysis. When evaluating data, these may be analysed qualitatively if no pooling of data is possible (if, for example end points vary widely from one trial to another). Interpretation of data then relies on a "vote-counting" of positive and negative results, which may take authors' (or reviewers') conclusions into consideration, but it should also include a quality and validity assessment of the individual trials.[3] A *qualitative* systematic review is a powerful tool to decide *whether* an intervention works. If data are combinable, they may be pooled and analysed in a meta-analysis, using the same scientific rigour, to provide a numerical or statistical output. This quantitative approach summarises the results, provides an estimate of the size of the effect, and helps to resolve disparities between conflicting studies. Such a *quantitative* systematic review that includes a meta-analysis is thus a powerful tool to inform us on *how well* the intervention works.

In reality, the process of performing and interpreting systematic reviews on postoperative pain control is often challenged through several issues. In single-dose analgesic trials, which mainly include patients undergoing minor surgical procedures (such as dental extraction), a single end point, for instance pain relief (which may be converted to a number needed to treat to achieve at least 50% pain relief), may be extracted (Chapter 4). However, contrary to single-dose analgesic trials, the main problem in the systematic review process when facing trials of other postoperative pain treatments is the lack of one common denominator. Pain relief will most often be evaluated with at least two measures: a pain assessment and a recording of rescue analgesic.

Pain may be reported as pain intensity or pain relief; both are usually reported as scores. Most often, assessments are made not only by the use of a visual analogue scale, but also by using a four- or five-point verbal rating scale, or by other scales, which may not be universally interchangeable. *Consumption of supplemental (or rescue) analgesics* may include a variety of analgesics such as opioids, non-opioids (for instance, paracetamol or non-steroidal inflammatory drugs), or local anaesthetics, etc. Furthermore, the analgesic consumption may be recorded in a number of ways – for example, in milligrams, in milligrams per kg bodyweight, or in number of dosages, each measured during time intervals, which may also vary. Finally, *time to first analgesic request* may be an end point, the relevance of which depends on the issue in question.

Thus, trials of postoperative pain treatment are often characterised by a large variety of end points that are not necessarily combinable. Therefore, even if data on, for instance, pain intensity scores allow a quantitative analysis, it is rarely possible to end up with one single estimate of the size of the effect of an analgesic; all relevant end points need to be considered in the overall synthesis and interpretation of the results.

Objective

The aim of this chapter was to provide an overview of the information that has become available through systematic reviews of *peripheral postoperative pain control*. We have chosen this subject among other possible topics on postoperative pain control because a considerable amount of research has been done on it during the past decade and because it is an area that has been well covered by several systematic reviews. A second aim was, from the clinical point of view, to critically appraise the soundness of the questions asked and answers provided, and to discuss the clinical utility of these (did these systematic reviews actually increase our knowledge of peripheral postoperative pain control?).

Methods

Published systematic reviews of peripheral treatment of postoperative pain were sought, without language restriction, in electronic databases (Medline, Cochrane Library), a web address (http://www.hcuge.ch/anesthesie/anglais/evidence/arevusyst.htm), relevant papers,[4] and books,[5,6] and by hand-searching locally available anaesthesia journals. Search terms included "systematic review", "meta-analysis", "audit", "postoperative pain", and "postoperative analgesia". We restricted our search to papers published up to the end of 2002. A review was considered *systematic* if it included a methods section with a clear question, a thorough systematic search strategy, definition of inclusion and exclusion criteria, and a structured data-handling and synthesis.[1]

Our main focus was on trials of drug interventions for peripheral postoperative pain treatment. From each systematic review, information was extracted on the covered setting, the question asked, the comparator for the intervention, the number of original trials and patients reviewed, the type of surgical procedures studied, answers provided on efficacy, and adverse effects. Furthermore, each systematic review was scored for quality using the Overview Quality Assessment Questionnaire (OQAQ).[7,8] The OQAQ is a validated checklist that asks nine questions on the methodological quality of the review. It does not measure literary quality, importance, relevance, originality, or other attributes of the reviews. The maximum possible OQAQ score for a given review is 7, indicating minimal flaws only. The minimal score is 1, indicating extensive flaws. Although additional valid evidence on a particular intervention may be available from individual randomised controlled trials, it is not included here unless it has been included in a systematic review.

59

Results

Retrieved systematic reviews

Fifty-eight systematic reviews dealing with issues of postoperative pain treatment were identified. Almost half of these were on single-dose analgesics (mainly oral), which are dealt with in another chapter (Chapter 4). Thirteen were systematic reviews on peripheral postoperative pain treatment.[9–21] Two of these were Cochrane reviews.[11,20] The systematic reviews covered incisional treatment,[9–14] intra-articular treatment,[13,15–19] and some aspects of nerve blocks.[12,13,20,21] The OQAQ scores ranged from 5 to 7 (Tables 5.1–5.3).

Incisional treatment and wound infiltration

Incisional local anaesthetics

Although widely used, local anaesthetic wound infiltration after abdominal operations showed only consistently improved analgesia in trials of inguinal hernia repair (Table 5.1).[9] The improvement could not be quantified due to the variety in end points. It was, however, judged to be clinically relevant but of short duration, which corresponded to the pharmacological duration of action of the local anaesthetics. Despite numerous trials, there was only weak or a lack of evidence (a lack of combinable data) for any clinically important effect for most other abdominal procedures.[9] However, in several trials, inadequate dosing and technique of local anaesthetic administration may partly explain the negative results.

Local anaesthetic port-site infiltration in diagnostic and operative gynaecological laparoscopy, cholecystectomy, and laparoscopic hernia repair did show an effect in at least one pain measurement in three of eight trials only.[10] Thus, these data did not provide evidence for a clinically worthwhile benefit from the intervention *per se* (Table 5.1). Furthermore, evidence was encountered for a statistically significant but clinically questionable effect from intraperitoneal infiltration with local anaesthetics after laparoscopic surgery.[10]

Perioperative local anaesthetic infiltration of the tonsillar bed was not shown to improve postoperative pain control after tonsillectomy in any trial that was included in a systematic review.[11] However, this conclusion was based on a few studies of small size and needs to be confirmed with further trials (Table 5.1).

No statistically significant or clinically worthwhile difference emerged in a meta-analysis on the effect of wound infiltration with local anaesthetics on pulmonary function after surgery (Table 5.1).[14]

Table 5.1 Overview of systematic reviews of peripheral postoperative pain treatment: incisional treatment

Reference	OQAQ score	Specific intervention	Design of systematic review/trials reviewed	No of trials/ patients included	Result	Implications for clinical practice	Implications for future research
Møiniche et al. 1998[9]	6	Local anaesthetic wound infiltration after open abdominal operation	Qualitative/ DB-RCT	26/1211	Except for herniotomy, there is a lack of evidence/ data for clinically important effects in most abdominal procedures	Seems to be a valuable technique for minor superficial procedures	Further trials of other minor procedures may verify benefit of method
Møiniche et al. 2000[10]	7	Local anaesthetic port-site infiltration after laparoscopy	Qualitative and quantitative/ DB-RCT	8/465	In three of eight trials analgesia was clinically improved, but questionable; WMD of VAS scores NS between treatment groups (95% CI −9 to 1)	Use of method per se of limited value	Future trials should be pharmacokinetic studies of combined large-dose, somato-visceral local anaesthetic block
Hollis et al. 1999[11]	6	Local anaesthetic infiltration for tonsillectomy	Qualitative/ DB-RCT	6/284	No documented effect in any of the few available trials	Method does not seem to provide additional benefit	No urgent need for further trials. Doubtful if more trials will change overall negative result

(Continued)

Table 5.1 (Continued)

Reference	OQAQ score	Specific intervention	Design of systematic review/trials reviewed	No of trials/ patients included	Result	Implications for clinical practice	Implications for future research
Ballantyne et al. 1998[14]	5	Effect of wound infiltration on pulmonary outcome	Qualitative/RCT	7/729	No documented effect	Considerations of pulmonary outcome is not an issue with wound infiltration	No need for further studies with respect to effect on pulmonary outcome of wound infiltration
Rømsing et al. 2000[13]	7	Wound infiltration with NSAID	Qualitative/ DB-RCT	7/324	No evidence for a peripheral analgesic effect	Method will provide no additional benefit	No urgent need for further trials. Doubtful if further research will change overall negative results
Picard et al. 1997[12]	7	Peripheral opioids (all except intra-articular) including incisional opioids	Qualitative/ DB-RCT	26/952	No evidence for a peripheral analgesic effect of incisional opioids (and plexus block, Bier's block, and other sites)	Method will provide no additional benefit	Trials without a systemic active control and placebo will not provide evidence for a peripheral effect nor ensure sensitivity of trial

DB = double-blind; CI = confidence interval; IA = intra-articular; NS = non-significant; OQAQ = Overview Quality Assessment Questionnaire; RCT = randomised controlled trial; VAS = visual analogue scale; WMD = weighted mean difference

Table 5.2 Overview of systematic reviews of peripheral postoperative pain treatment: intra-articular treatment of the knee

Reference	OQAQ score	Specific intervention	Design of systematic review/trials reviewed	No of trials/patients included	Result	Implications for clinical practice	Implications for future research
Møiniche et al. 1999[15]	7	IA local anaesthetic instillation after arthroscopic procedures	Qualitative and quantitative/DB-RCT	20/895	Weak evidence for small-to-moderate and short-lasting effect	Method may provide short-lasting but still clinically relevant pain relief in day-case surgery	No need for further trials on local anaesthetics alone, but rather on IA multimodal regimens. Owing to sensitivity reasons the pain model should cause a certain level of pain
Kalso et al. 1997[16]	6	IA morphine after arthroscopic procedures	Qualitative/DB-RCT	15/779 (only four RCTs with systemic control)	Overall result indicates some prolonged, rather than early, effect in pain intensity and analgesic consumption	Systematic reviews are in agreement overall regarding an especially late analgesic effect, which may be clinically relevant in day-case surgery	Only trials with an adequate level of pain in control group can be considered sensitive (no pain, no gain). Further trials including systemic opioid control and placebo are needed to document a *peripheral* effect and ensure sensitivity of trial

(Continued)

Table 5.2 (Continued)

Reference	OQAQ score	Specific intervention	Design of systematic review/trials reviewed	No of trials/ patients included	Result	Implications for clinical practice	Implications for future research
Meiser et al. 1997[17]	4	IA opioids after arthroscopic procedures	Qualitative/ DB-RCT	34/1950 (only six RCTs with systemic control)	A small dose of IA morphine seems to exert a late, rather than early, analgesic effect		
Gupta et al. 2001[18]	7	IA morphine after arthroscopic procedures	Qualitative and quantitative/ DB-RCT	28/1800 (only five RCTs with systemic control)	WMD of VAS scores improved 12–17 mm compared with placebo. Analgesic consumption was reduced in 6 of 13 positive trials. Result from comparisons with systemic control equivocal		
Kalso et al. 2002[19]	7	IA morphine after arthroscopic procedures	Qualitative/ DB-RCT	28/1103 (only three RCTs with systemic control)	10 of 13 sensitive trials showed improved analgesia up to 24 hours after surgery compared with placebo Systemic control comparisons negative		

(Continued)

Table 5.2 (*Continued*)

Reference	OQAQ score	Specific intervention	Design of systematic review/trials reviewed	No of trials/ patients included	Result	Implications for clinical practice	Implications for future research
Rømsing et al. 2000[13]	7	IA NSAID after arthroscopic procedures	Qualitative and quantitative/ DB-RCT	7/370 (only three RCTs with systemic control)	Based on three available RCTs that included a systemic control. Indication of a clinically relevant peripheral analgesic effect	Use of method should await confirmation of data	Need for further trials to document promising preliminary results. Trials without a systemic active control and placebo will not provide evidence for a peripheral effect and ensure sensitivity of trial

DB = double-blind; IA = intra-articular; OQAQ = Overview Quality Assessment Questionnaire; RCT = randomised controlled trial; VAS = visual analogue scale; WMD = weighted mean difference

Table 5.3 Overview of systematic reviews of peripheral postoperative pain treatment: peripheral block

Reference	OQAQ score	Specific intervention	Design of systematic review/trials reviewed	No of trials/ patients included	Result	Implications for clinical practice	Implications for future research
Parker et al. 1999[20]	7	Subcostal, lateral cutaneous, femoral, triple, psoas local anaesthetic block for hip fractures	Qualitative/RCT or quasi-RCT	6/229	Improved pain control in the immediate postoperative period Lack of data to show an associated clinical benefit	Nerve blocks inserted peri-operatively reduce the need for parenteral analgesics	Large-scale trials of *individual methods* needed to confirm results Future trials should use validated pain scales and analgesic consumption as endpoints
Rømsing et al. 2000[13]	7	NSAID as a component of IV regional anaesthesia	Qualitative and quantitative/ DB-RCT	3/130	Improved pain control compared with placebo Only one comparison with systemic control	Use of methods should await further trials	Trials without a systemic active control and placebo will not provide evidence for a peripheral effect and ensure sensitivity of trial
Murphy et al. 2000[21]	6	Adjuncts for peripheral nerve blocks	Qualitative/ DB-RCT	17/796	No firm evidence for improved analgesia with brachial plexus block adjuncts	Use of method in preference to systemic treatment not supported	No need for further trials on perineural adjunct opioid Trials without a systemic active

(Continued)

Table 5.3 *(Continued)*

Reference	OQAQ score	Specific intervention	Design of systematic review/trials reviewed	No of trials/ patients included	Result	Implications for clinical practice	Implications for future research
					(opioids and clonidine) over systemic administration. Only five trials included systemic control		control and placebo will not provide evidence for a peripheral effect and ensure sensitivity of trial
Picard et al. 1997[12]	7	Peripheral opioids (all except intra-articular)	Qualitative/ RCT	26/952	No evidence for a clinically relevant analgesic effect of peripheral opioids in plexus block, Bier's block, or other perineural block	Method will provide no additional benefit	No need for further trials

DB = double-blind; IV = intravenous; OQAQ = Overview Quality Assessment Questionnaire; RCT = randomised controlled trial

Peripheral opioids (including incisional but excluding intra-articular)

Peripheral opioids may have a peripheral analgesic effect in inflamed tissues. In only one of five clinical trials, wound infiltration with opioids, or intraperitoneal or intrapleural application of opioids, was associated with a statistically significant reduction in pain.[12] This difference was not judged to be clinically relevant by the authors of the review. Even though data on incisional opioid administration are sparse, they suggest, together with data on other peripheral application of opioids (all except intraarticular, see below), that there is no clinically relevant analgesic effect of peripheral opioids as compared with systemic administration in the acute pain setting (Table 5.1).

Incisional NSAIDs

Local administration of NSAIDs in order to achieve a peripheral effect may seem an attractive method, as systemic concentrations – and thus, NSAID-related adverse effects – would be reduced. Quantitative and qualitative analysis of data from seven randomised controlled trials did not, however, support the view that pain relief may be improved with wound infiltration with NSAIDs as compared with systemic NSAID administration;[13] this technique cannot be recommended (Table 5.1).

Intra-articular treatment

Intra-articular local anaesthetics

Intra-articular local anaesthetic instillation, a technique commonly used by many orthopaedic surgeons, has been shown to reduce postoperative pain after arthroscopic surgery. However, the evidence was not compelling as only 12 of 20 studies showed better pain relief with intra-articular local anaesthetics.[15] The effect was best documented in trials in which patients had a certain level of pain – that is, more than moderate pain (> 30 mm VAS (visual analogue scale)) – in the placebo group (Table 5.2).[15] Only quantitative analysis of VAS scores revealed a modest effect (weighted mean difference, 11 mm) in favour of the treatment. It is difficult, therefore, to interpret precisely how well the interventions worked, given that the majority of trials also reported on analgesic consumption. Overall, the effect seemed to be moderate and of short duration only; this, however, may still be of clinical importance in day-case surgery.[15]

Intra-articular opioids

Four systematic reviews of intra-articular opioids for pain relief after arthroscopic surgery have been published (Table 5.2).[16–19] The systematic reviews share some important features, although they differ somewhat in study design and conclusions reached. The main problem when analysing the effect of intra-articular opioids is methodological. Analgesic efficacy may depend on several factors: the type of surgical procedure that is performed (whether the procedure causes enough inflammation in the knee and enough postoperative pain); the anaesthetic technique that is used for surgery (regional versus general); the dose of morphine; and the method of pain assessment (pain at rest versus pain during activity, and early pain versus late pain after surgery). In the most recent review,[19] emphasis was therefore placed on study sensitivity. For a study to be sensitive, it is paramount that there is a minimal amount of pain, as it is impossible to measure pain relief if pain is absent or only mild.

Overall, these systematic reviews can be interpreted as evidence that intra-articular morphine causes a minor improvement in pain relief after surgical procedures but not after diagnostic procedures, compared with placebo. The effect starts early and has a surprisingly long duration – up to 24 hours after surgery. The latter may be explained by the proportionally large depot of intra-articular morphine, which may be available for hours while inflammation and peripheral opioid receptors develop in the knee joint. A dose of 5 mg of morphine seems to be more effective than 1 mg.[19] However, even though the long duration of action may indicate a peripheral analgesic effect, there is a lack of direct evidence for a peripheral effect compared with a systemic analgesic effect.[16-19] Only a few trials included a systemic opioid control, and only a minority of those showed improved pain relief with peripheral compared with systemic treatment. Hence, a systemic effect of intra-articular opioid cannot be excluded. The clinical relevance and site of action of the intervention are difficult to evaluate. The technique may indeed be worthwhile if, for example, sending outpatients home with a prescription of morphine can be avoided.

Intra-articular NSAIDs

Only three trials compared intra-articular with systemic NSAID treatment; there seemed to be some indication of a clinically relevant peripheral mediated action of intra-articular NSAIDs.[13] These results, which are based on only about 100 patients receiving intra-articular NSAIDs, need to be confirmed (Table 5.2).

Nerve blocks

Nerve blocks (subcostal, lateral cutaneous, femoral, triple, psoas) for hip fractures

Evidence from six randomised or pseudo-randomised trials showed a reduction in the quantity of parenteral or oral analgesic demands (rescue analgesics) in the immediate postoperative period when nerve blocks were used.[20] However, none of the trials had a large enough number of patients to show whether this reduction in analgesic use was associated with any clinical benefit (Table 5.3).

Adjuncts for nerve blocks

Opioids or non-opioids may be added to a brachial plexus block, other perineural blocks, or a Bier's block with local anaesthetics to improve intra-operative and postoperative analgesia. Two systematic reviews, which differed somewhat in inclusion criteria and interpretation of studies, have examined the literature regarding this issue (Table 5.3).[12,21]

Of 15 studies that tested opioids, six reported a statistically significant benefit in pain relief.[12,21] This difference was, however, only rarely judged to be clinically relevant by the authors of the reviews. Furthermore, only two of four trials that included a systemic opioid control showed improved analgesia with the brachial plexus administration of the opioid. In addition, there was no reduction in opioid-related adverse effects with the peripheral administration of opioids.[21] Trials of lower quality were more likely to report increased efficacy with peripheral opioids.[12]

Of six studies that tested clonidine, five found that analgesia was improved. However, only one study included a systemic clonidine control group.[21] There is, therefore, no convincing evidence from these systematic reviews that adjunct opioids or non-opioid (clonidine) analgesics in brachial plexus or other perineural blocks are of any benefit compared with the systemic treatment.

Finally, there was a lack of data regarding the use of NSAIDs as a component of a Bier's block compared with systemic NSAID administration.[13]

Discussion

Taken together, evidence from systematic reviews supported only the use of wound infiltration with local anaesthetics in hernia repair and possibly other minor superficial surgical procedures. With respect to wound infiltration with opioids and NSAIDs, no evidence for any effect was found when compared with systemic administration.

Evidence on intra-articular treatment was generally positive, showing improved postoperative pain relief with intra-articular local anaesthetics and opioid. The individual time profile for maximum pain relief may favour a combination of these drugs. At first sight there is no direct evidence for a local (peripheral) action of intra-articular morphine. This will be discussed further below. The promising data on intra-articular NSAIDs should be confirmed before these drugs are recommended for routine use.

Peripheral nerve blocks reduce the need for other analgesics after hip fracture, but evidence for any clinical benefit for the patient is not yet available. Furthermore, more data on the individual types of nerve blocks are needed before final recommendations can be made. Finally, opioid or non-opioid analgesics in peripheral nerve blocks provide no additional benefit over systemic administration.

These systematic reviews provide several answers to a number of questions relating to interventions – for example, for what peripheral analgesic method is there a scientific basis? What method should be discarded? Or, for what method are further data needed? Although most of the reviews could determine whether or not an intervention worked, few (if any) were able to give an overall estimate of the size of the effect of the analgesic intervention. Most analyses were performed as qualitative reviews, as there was a large variety in end points that could not be combined; some included a quantitative analysis (a meta-analysis), but only for one of several end points (typically, VAS pain scores). Only few data were provided on the impact of the interventions on, for instance, immediate recovery or various convalescence measures. Furthermore, no comparisons with other analgesics or analgesic techniques were provided; such direct comparisons are helpful in deciding whether an invasive intervention is worth its effort, or if similar analgesia might be achieved with simple systemic treatment. It remains difficult to place those peripheral analgesic techniques that seemed to provide effective pain control into a hierarchy of analgesic treatments. Finally, only little insight on potential adverse effects or risks could be extracted from the systematic reviews. Thus, the clinical utility remains difficult to evaluate.

The reviews were generally of a high quality, according to the Overview Quality Assessment Questionnaire (OQAQ). The questionnaire tests whether formal methodology is performed adequately. It has previously shown that systematic reviews of low quality are more likely to produce positive conclusions than reviews of high quality.[8] However, it must be realised that the questionnaire does not measure importance, relevance, or soundness of the questions asked, or even further attributes of a systematic review. Furthermore, we found the OQAQ scoring to be too flexible and not easy to use. The value of this questionnaire may therefore be disputed. As another option, systematic reviews may be evaluated by using "The Quality of Reporting of Meta-analyses (QUOROM) statement",[22] which, although it is a guideline for conducting and reporting systematic reviews, may also be used to evaluate the quality of those reviews.

A lesson learned from these systematic reviews concerns some methodological issues. When evaluating a local effect of peripherally

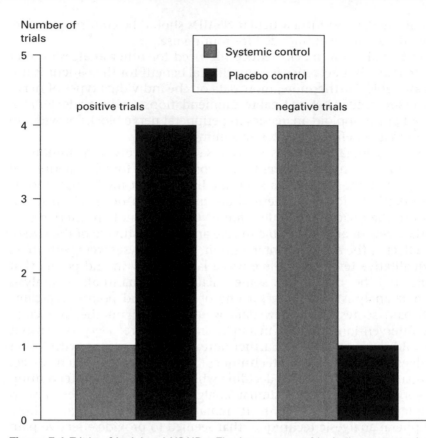

Figure 5.1 Trials of incisional NSAIDs. The importance of including a systemic control to ensure a local rather than systemic effect of peripherally applied analgesics. The number of positive and negative studies (evaluated 1–2 hours postoperatively) in which incisional NSAIDs were compared with placebo or with systemic NSAIDs is shown. Trials comparing incisional NSAIDs with placebo were generally positive, whereas trials comparing incisional NSAIDs with systemic NSAIDs were generally negative. Thus, trials without a systemic control may measure a systemic effect of the locally applied NSAID, and cannot provide evidence for a local effect. Adapted from[13]

administered analgesics such as opioids or NSAIDs, it is important to control for a systemic effect. This can be done by including a systemic control group. A systematic review of wound infiltration with NSAIDs found that comparisons with placebo were generally in favour of the peripheral NSAID, whereas most trials with a systemic control group were negative[13] (Figure 5.1). This probably reflects the fact that peripherally applied NSAIDs are more analgesic than no treatment (or a placebo), but that this effect may well be mediated through a central or a peripheral action. Thus, trials without a systemic control group

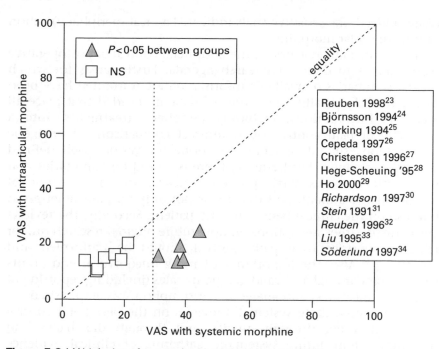

Figure 5.2 L'Abbé plot of mean visual analogue scale (VAS) pain scores for intra-articular versus systemic morphine control. Each point represents an individual trial. Triangles represent trials with statistical significance in VAS pain scores in the early (2–6 hours) postoperative period; squares are trials with no statistical significance between treatment groups. Only trials on the right-hand side of the horizontal dotted line (placed at 30 mm VAS in systemic controls) reported enough pain to be considered sensitive assays ("no pain, no gain"[19]). Names at the right-hand side of the graph indicate trials (references). Names in italics indicate trials with a significant difference in favour of the intra-articular treatment

should not be regarded as valid assays to evaluate the peripheral effect of analgesics.

Another lesson learnt was that the sensitivity of the studies was very important. If there is only little pain it may be impossible to detect an improvement or, as expressed by Kalso,[19] if there is no pain there is no gain. We performed an updated search on trials of intra-articular morphine and plotted the results on a L'Abbé plot for illustration. In 12 trials of intra-articular versus systemic morphine,[23-34] only five trials[30-34] showed significantly improved pain relief with intra-articular treatment two to six hours postoperatively. However, these were the only trials with an adequate level of pain (> 30 mm VAS in the control group) and thus the only trials that could be considered as being sensitive (Figure 5.2). So, if applying a simple "vote counting" of positive and negative trials, the insensitive trials may blur the overall result. Indeed, the sensitive trials indicated a local (peripheral) action of intra-articular morphine.

These systematic reviews on the peripheral control of postoperative pain help us to define a research agenda. Firstly, areas for which further summaries of available information are warranted have been highlighted. Especially, summaries of data are needed that place all analgesic interventions, including peripheral treatments, into a hierarchy of pain control. Such indirect comparisons of analgesic interventions should preferably be done for various well defined surgical procedures. Furthermore, there is a need for summaries that place interventions with proven efficacy, in the context of multimodal treatment, and that focus not only on pain relief *per se* but also on the clinical benefit for the patient. Secondly, the reviews emphasised earlier suggestions on how future original research on, for instance, postoperative pain control should be performed and reported.[35,36] Also, the importance of using unequivocal end points such as standardised and validated pain scales (including reporting of dispersion measures) and analgesic consumption was emphasised.

In conclusion, these systematic reviews on the peripheral control of pain indicate, through quality and through drawbacks and limitations, how future systematic gathering of clinical evidence of postoperative pain treatment should continue.

References

1. Cook DJ, Sackett DL, Spitzer WO. Methodologic guidelines for systematic reviews of randomised control trials in health care from the Potsdam Consultation on Meta-Analysis. *J Clin Epidemiol* 1995;**48**:167–71.
2. Rosenberg W, Donald A. Evidence based medicine: an approach to clinical problem-solving. *BMJ* 1995;**310**:1122–6.
3. Smith LA, Oldman AD, McQuay HJ, Moore RA. Teasing apart quality and validity in systematic reviews: an example from acupuncture trials in chronic neck and back pain. *Pain* 2000;**86**:119–32.
4. Choi PTL, Halpern SH, Malik N, Jadad AR, Tramèr M, Walder B. Examining the evidence in anesthesia literature: a critical appraisal of systematic reviews. *Anesth Analg* 2001;**92**:700–9.
5. Tramèr MR. Appendix: Systematic reviews relevant to anaesthetists. In: Tramèr MR, ed. *An evidence based resource in anaesthesia and analgesia*. London: BMJ Books, 2000;197–218.
6. McQuay HJ, Moore RA. Existing systematic reviews. In: McQuay HJ, Moore RA, eds. *An evidence-based resource for pain relief*. New York: Oxford University Press, 1998;39–49.
7. Oxman AD, Guyatt GH. Validation of an index of the quality of review articles. *J Clin Epidemiol* 1991;**44**:1271–8.
8. Jadad AR, McQuay HJ. Meta-analyses to evaluate analgesic interventions: a systematic qualitative review of their methodology. *J Clin Epidemiol* 1996;**49**:235–43.
9. Møiniche S, Mikkelsen S, Wetterslev J, Dahl JB. A qualitative systematic review of incisional local anaesthesia for postoperative pain relief after abdominal operations. *Br J Anaesth* 1998;**81**:377–83.

10. Møiniche S, Jørgensen H, Wetterslev J, Dahl JB. Local anesthetic infiltration for postoperative pain relief after laparoscopy: a qualitative and quantitative systematic review of intraperitoneal, port-site infiltration and mesosalpinx block. *Anesth Analg* 2000;**90**:899–912.
11. Hollis LJ, Burton MJ, Millar JM. Perioperative local anaesthesia for reducing pain following tonsillectomy (Cochrane Review). In: Cochrane Collaboration. *Cochrane Library*. Issue 4. Oxford: Update Software, 2002.
12. Picard PR, Tramèr MR, McQuay HJ, Moore RA. Analgesic efficacy of peripheral opioids (all except intraarticular): a qualitative systematic review of randomised controlled trials. *Pain* 1997;**72**:309–18.
13. Rømsing J, Møiniche S, Østergaard D, Dahl JB. Local infiltration with NSAIDs for postoperative analgesia: evidence for a peripheral analgesic action. *Acta Anaesthesiol Scand* 2000;**44**:672–83.
14. Ballantyne JC, Carr DB, deFerranti S, *et al*. The comparative effects of postoperative analgesic therapies on pulmonary outcome: cumulative meta-analyses of randomized, controlled trials. *Anesth Analg* 1998;**86**:598–612.
15. Møiniche S, Mikkelsen S, Wetterslev J, Dahl JB. A systematic review of intraarticular local anesthesia for postoperative pain relief after arthroscopic knee surgery. *Reg Anesth Pain Med* 1999;**24**:430–7.
16. Kalso E, Tramèr MR, Carroll D, McQuay HJ, Moore RA. Pain relief from intraarticular morphine after knee surgery: a qualitative systematic review. *Pain* 1997;**71**:127–34.
17. Meiser A, Laubenthal H. Klinische Studien zur peripheren Wirksamkeit von Opioiden nach Kniegelenk-Operationen. *Anaesthesist* 1997;**46**:867–79.
18. Gupta A, Bodein L, Holmström, Berggren L. A systematic review of the peripheral analgesic effects of intraarticular morphine. *Anesth Analg* 2001;**93**:761–70.
19. Kalso E, Smith L, McQuay HJ, Moore RA. No pain, no gain: clinical excellence and scientific rigour – lessons learned from IA morphine. *Pain* 2002;**98**:269–75.
20. Parker MJ, Griffiths R, Appadu BN. Nerve blocks (subcostal, lateral cutaneous, femoral, triple, psoas) for hip fractures (Cochrane Review). In: Cochrane Collaboration. *Cochrane Library*. Issue 4. Oxford: Update Software, 2002.
21. Murphy DB, McCartney CJ, Chan VW. Novel analgesic adjuncts for brachial plexus block: a systematic review. *Anesth Analg* 2000;**90**:1122–8.
22. Moher D, Cook DJ, Eastwood S, Olkin I, Rennie D, Stroup DF. Improving the quality of reports of meta-analyses of randomised controlled trials: the QUOROM statement. Quality of Reporting of Meta-analyses. *Lancet* 1999;**354**: 1896–900.
23. Reuben SS, Steinberg RB, Cohen MA, Kilaru PA, Gibson CS. Intraarticular morphine in the multimodal analgesic management of postoperative pain after ambulatory anterior cruciate ligament repair. *Anesth Analg* 1998;**86**:374–8.
24. Björnsson A, Gupta A, Vegfors M, Lennmarken C, Sjöberg F. Intraarticular morphine for postoperative analgesia following knee arthoscopy. *Reg Anesth* 1994;**19**:104–8.
25. Dierking GW, Østergaard HT, Dissing CK, Kristensen JE, Dahl JB. Analgesic effect of intraarticular morphine after arthroscopic meniscectomy. *Anaesthesia* 1994;**49**:627–9.
26. Cepeda MS, Uribe C, Betancourt J, Rugeles J, Carr DB. Pain relief after knee arthroscopy: intraarticular morphine, intraarticular bupivacaine, or subcutaneous morphine? *Reg Anesth* 1997;**22**:233–8.
27. Christensen O, Christensen P, Sonnenschein C, Nielsen PR, Jacobsen S. Analgesic effect of intraarticular morphine: a controlled, randomised and double-blind study. *Acta Anaesthesiol Scand* 1996;**40**:842–6.
28. Hege-Scheuing G, Michaelsen K, Bühler A, Kustermann J, Seeling W. Analgesie durch intraartikuläres Morphin nach Kniegelenksarthroskopien? *Anaesthesist* 1995;**44**:351–8.
29. Ho ST, Wang JJ, Tang JJS, Liaw WL, Ho CM. Pain relief after arthroscopic knee surgery: intravenous morphine, epidural morphine, and intraarticular morphine. *Clin J Pain* 2000;**16**:105–9.
30. Richardson MD, Bjorksten AR, Hart JAL, McCullough K. The efficacy of intraarticular morphine for postoperative knee arthroscopy analgesia. *Arthroscopy* 1997;**13**:584–9.
31. Stein C, Comisel K, Haimeri E, *et al*. Analgesic effect of intraarticular morphine after arthroscopic knee surgery. *N Engl J Med* 1991;**325**:1123–6.

32. Reuben SS, Connelly NR. Postarthroscopic meniscus repair analgesia with intraarticular ketorolac or morphine. *Anesth Analg* 1996;**82**:1036–9.
33. Liu K, Wang JJ, Ho St, Liaw WJ, Chia YY. Opioid in peripheral analgesia: intraarticular morphine for pain control after arthroscopic knee surgery. *Acta Anaesthesiol Sin* 1995;**33**:217–21.
34. Söderlund A, Westman L, Ersmark H, Eriksson E, Valentin A, Ekblom A. Analgesia following arthroscopy: a comparison of intraarticular morphine, pethidine and fentanyl. *Acta Anaesthesiol Scand* 1997;**41**:6–11.
35. Begg C, Cho M, Eastwood S, *et al.* Improving the quality of reporting of randomized controlled trials: the CONSORT statement. *JAMA* 1996;**276**:637–9.
36. Moher D, Schulz KF, Altman DG. The CONSORT statement: revised recommendations for improving the quality of reports of parallel-group randomised trials. *Lancet* 2001;**357**:1191–4.

6: Epidural analgesia for labour and delivery

STEPHEN HALPERN, BARBARA LEIGHTON

Epidural analgesia effectively relieves labour pain and is often chosen by parturients because of the known efficacy of the technique. However, some authors express concern about potential side effects of epidural analgesia on the progress of labour, the fetus, and the newborn child. Over the past 20 years, new methods of administration and maintenance of epidural analgesia have been described and studied. Some of these innovations have improved outcomes, whereas others have not. In this chapter we will review the effects of epidural analgesia on maternal and neonatal outcomes. We will then discuss the more important innovations in the delivery of epidural labour analgesia. Some of this information is available in published systematic reviews and meta-analyses. These have been updated with additional information from electronic searches of the literature, most recently on 15 January 2003.

Epidural analgesia and the progress of labour

Effect of epidural labour analgesia on the rates of caesarean and instrumented vaginal delivery

Three types of studies have been reported to measure the effect of epidural analgesia on the incidence of caesarean delivery: cohort observational studies (prospective and retrospective), randomised controlled trials in which epidural analgesia is compared with parenteral opioids, and observational studies in which a prospective cohort is compared with a retrospective cohort after an epidural service has been instituted ("before and after" studies). Each of these study designs has advantages and disadvantages. For ethical reasons, there have been no placebo controlled randomised trials.

Compared with other study designs, observational studies are inexpensive and can rapidly generate data on a large number of patients. These studies have shown a strong association between epidural analgesia and the incidence of caesarean section.[1] This association was present even when multivariate statistics were used in an attempt to control confounding variables.[2] The authors of these studies concluded that epidurals probably *caused* the negative outcomes, and one group suggested that this retrospective data be routinely discussed with patients in order to help them make an informed decision.[3] However, women who have a more painful latent phase of labour are more likely to have a dysfunctional labour, leading to requests for more analgesia and more obstetrical interventions.[4,5] Increased pain and prolonged latent phase are also the reasons that many patients choose to have epidural analgesia. Therefore, increased pain may be a marker for poor obstetric outcome, and these patients are more likely to request epidural analgesia. Data from observational studies are therefore not reliable and will not be considered further.

In many clinical scenarios, randomised controlled trials are considered to be the most rigorous evidence available to determine the effects of treatment. In this case, randomised trials are particularly difficult to perform because of the clear superiority of the analgesia in the epidural group compared with, for example, parenteral opioids. It is not possible to blind these studies. Because there is some subjectivity in deciding the need for and timing of caesarean or instrumented vaginal delivery for dystocia, knowledge of patient treatment group could introduce bias. Another problem is that women with strong feelings for or against epidural analgesia do not enrol in these trials. Because many women make this decision before the onset of labour, this eliminates a large fraction of parturients from study participation. This may reduce the applicability of the results to the general population. Finally, many patients "cross over" to the epidural group if they are assigned to the opioid group. If enough patients change groups, the randomisation may be threatened.

In spite of these difficulties, randomised allocation to epidural versus parenteral opioid labour analgesia was reported in 14 studies enrolling 4441 patients.[6-19] This is an update of a previous analysis.[20] The overall rate of caesarean delivery did not differ between the two groups (odds ratio (OR) 1·00, 95% confidence interval 0·78–1·27) (Figure 6.1). Other obstetrical outcomes and neonatal outcomes are shown in Table 6.1. The overall rate of instrumental vaginal delivery was higher in the epidural group than in the opioid group (2·05, 1·07–2·87; $P < 0.001$), but the incidence of instrumental delivery for dystocia was not. Maternal satisfaction and pain relief in the first and second stages of labour were better in epidural group patients. Fever (maternal temperature > 38°C) was more frequent in epidural group patients. There was no difference in the incidence of severe neonatal asphyxia as shown by umbilical artery cord gases. Measures such as the early Apgar scores and the need for naloxone favoured the use of epidural analgesia, reflecting the temporary effect of maternal opioids on the newborn (Table 6.1).

Study	Epidural n/N	Opiod n/N	OR (random) 95% CI	OR (random) 95% CI
Robinson (1) 1980[16]	0/28	0/30		Not estimable
Robinson (2) 1980[16]	0/17	0/18		Not estimable
Nikkola 1997[12]	0/10	0/10		Not estimable
Clark 1998[7]	15/156	22/162		0·68 (0·34, 1·36)
Sharma 1997[17]	13/358	16/357		0·80 (0·38, 1·70)
Sharma 2002[18]	16/226	20/233		0·81 (0·41, 1·61)
Howell 2001[8]	13/175	16/178		0·81 (0·38, 1·74)
Loughnan 2000[9]	36/304	40/310		0·91 (0·56, 1·47)
Muir 2000[11]	11/97	9/88		1·12 (0·44, 2·85)
Ramin 1995[15]	43/664	37/666		1·18 (0·75, 1·85)
Muir 1996[10]	3/28	2/22		1·20 (0·18, 7·89)
Philipsen (1989[13], 1990[14])	10/57	6/54		1·70 (0·57, 5·06)
Bofill 1997[6]	5/49	3/51		1·82 (0·41, 8·06)
Thorp 1993[19]	12/48	1/45		14·67 (1·82, 118·22)
Total (95% CI)	177/2217	172/2224		1·00 (0·78, 1·27)

Test for overall effect Z = 0·02 (P = 0·98)

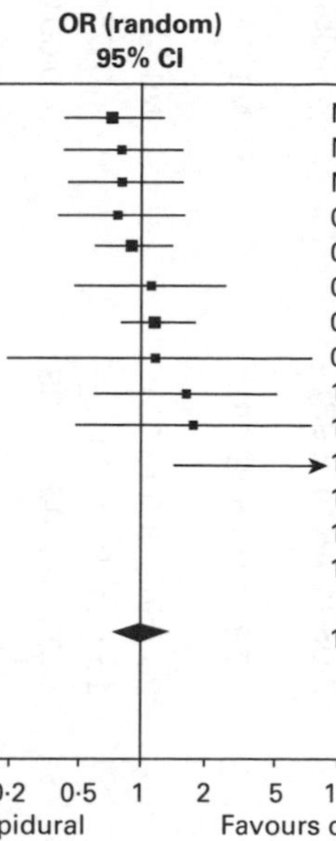

0·1 0·2 0·5 1 2 5 10
Favours epidural   Favours opioid

Figure 6.1 Epidural versus parenteral opioid analgesia for labour. The individual and pooled odds ratios (OR) and 95% confidence intervals (CI) for caesarean section are shown. The size of each box is proportional to the contribution of the study to the pooled results. There was no difference in the incidence of caesarean section between the groups (OR = 1·00)

In an attempt to avoid some of the problems encountered in randomised controlled trials, some investigators have studied institutions that did not offer epidural analgesia on the labour floor and which then, over a brief period of time, introduced epidural analgesia into practice. Although many factors can threaten the validity of this design (such as changes in practice or personnel over the study period), when compared with randomised controlled trials, there are some advantages. This approach eliminates the problem of patients' choosing epidural analgesia when assigned to another treatment group because epidural analgesia was not available. Similarly, these studies (provided that the data are collected in a comprehensive and reliable manner) are more applicable to the full population. Since 1990, there have been five published studies that have done this.[21–25] As can be seen in Figure 6.2, there was no appreciable change in the caesarean section rate, even with a large incremental change in the epidural rate. Furthermore, a recent meta-analysis of published and unpublished data confirmed that there was no increase in the incidence of forceps deliveries caused by the increased availability of epidural analgesia.[26]

Table 6.1 Epidural versus parenteral opioid analgesia: maternal neonatal outcomes

Outcome	No of studies included	Epidural n/N or N	Opioid n/N or N	Odds ratio or weighted mean difference (95% confidence interval)	P value
Maternal outcomes					
Instrumental vaginal delivery	11	344/1813	226/1840	2·08 (1·48 to 2·93)	< 0·05
Instrumental vaginal delivery for dystocia	3	39/538	23/542	1·53 (0·29 to 8·08)	NS
1st stage of labour (min)	7	1012	1050	26 min (−8·0 to 60)	NS
2nd stage of labour (min)	8	1068	1103	15 min (9 to 22)	< 0·05
Maternal pain – 1st stage of labour (VAS mm)	7	1017	1014	−40 mm (−42 to −38)	< 0·001
Maternal pain – 2nd stage of labour (VAS mm)	5	536	526	−29 mm (−38 to −21)	< 0·001
Maternal fever (> 38·0°C)	3	212/845	49/868	5·6 (4·0 to 7·8)	< 0·001
Satisfaction	6	128/951	340/968	0·27 (0·19 to 0·38)	< 0·001
Neonatal outcomes					
Apgar score < 7 at 1 min	10	49/1456	105/1477	0·4 (0·18 to 0·87)	0·02
Apgar score < 7 at 5 min	8	8/1273	15/1272	0·54 (0·23 to 1·26)	NS
Low umbilical artery pH	6	143/1025	173/1009	1·0 (0·18 to 5·44)	NS
Severe asphyxia: umbilical artery pH < 6·99	5	3/1083	3/1084	0·56 (0·15 to 2·17)	NS
Need for naloxone in the newborn	4	3/587	24/590	0·20 (0·10 to 0·44)	< 0·01

NS = not significant; VAS = visual analogue scale.

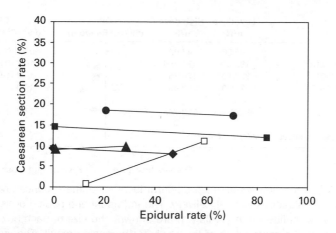

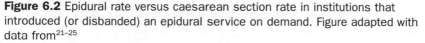

Figure 6.2 Epidural rate versus caesarean section rate in institutions that introduced (or disbanded) an epidural service on demand. Figure adapted with data from[21-25]

High-dose versus low-dose local analgesia and mode of delivery

If epidural analgesia influenced the mode of delivery, one would expect that high concentrations of local anaesthetic would have a greater influence than low concentrations. In the section above, we concluded that epidural analgesia does not lead to an increase in the caesarean section rate, although it may increase the forceps delivery rate when compared with opioid analgesia. However, in many of the studies cited, patients assigned to the opioid group found this form of analgesia inadequate and therefore "crossed over" to the epidural group. It is possible that those that crossed over represented a subset of the population that was at higher risk for forceps delivery. Furthermore, because the studies could not be blinded, the use of an epidural may have influenced the behaviour of the obstetricians. This was clearly stated in one of the studies, in which 85% of women in the epidural group who underwent forceps delivery did so for the purpose of resident training.[6]

Four randomised controlled trials have compared low concentrations (defined as < 0·125% bupivacaine) with higher concentrations.[27-30] Three of these[27,28,30] used a combined spinal–epidural technique to initiate analgesia. In total, 1344 patients received low concentrations of local anaesthetic and 748 received high concentrations. A meta-analysis of these studies found no difference in the incidence of caesarean section. However, there was a statistically significant increase in the incidence of forceps delivery and a corresponding reduction in the spontaneous delivery rate (Figure 6.3).[31] Notably,

Study	Low dose n/N	High dose n/N	OR (95% CI Random)	OR (95% CI Random)
Collis 1995[27]	46/98	47/99		0·98 (0·56, 1·71)
Nageotte 1997[30]	292/505	130/256		1·33 (0·98, 1·80)
COMET 2001[28]	300/701	124/353		1·38 (1·06, 1·80)
James 1998[29]	27/40	22/40		1·70 (0·68, 4·22)
Total (95% CI)	665/1344	323/748		1·32 (1·10, 1·59)

Test for overall effect z = −2·99 p = 0·003

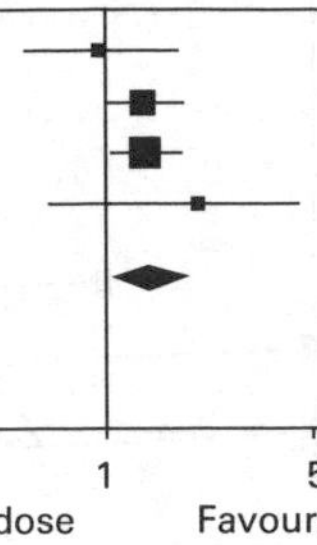

−1   −2   1   5   10
Favours low dose   Favours high dose

Figure 6.3 Effect of low versus high epidural local anaesthetic concentration on the rate of spontaneous vaginal delivery. The individual and pooled odds ratios (OR) with 95% confidence intervals (CI) are shown. The size of each box is proportional to the contribution of the study to the pooled result. The incidence of spontaneous vaginal delivery is higher in the low-dose group (OR = 1·32, P = 0·003)

there was no difference between any of the obstetrical outcomes in either of the studies that compared combined spinal–epidural analgesia with low-concentration labour epidural analgesia.[28,30] These observations support the contention that epidural analgesia may increase the rate of forceps delivery. However, the impact of this effect can be minimised by using low concentrations of local anaesthetic for initiation and maintenance of labour analgesia. Combined spinal–epidural analgesia appears to be no different from low-dose epidural analgesia with respect to mode of delivery.

Epidural analgesia and long-term back pain

Back pain after childbirth is common. In the absence of epidural analgesia, early studies estimate that the incidence of back pain within the first six days post partum is about 38%.[32] Whether or not long-term back pain is caused by epidural analgesia is controversial. In a large retrospective study, investigators surveyed patients who had delivered a baby in their institution within the previous nine years. Their results indicated that there was a strong association between epidural use and long-term back pain.[33] The authors concluded that this association was probably causal. However, retrospective studies concerning peripartum back pain are subject to important inaccuracy and potential biases. In particular, women are unable to consistently recall the magnitude of their back pain near the time of childbirth, when asked about it later. In a one-year follow-up study, Macarthur et al. found that only 56% of women accurately recalled the amount of

Table 6.2 Epidural analgesia and long-term back pain: characteristics of studies

Study	Design	Epidural (No)	Non-epidural (No)	Duration of follow up
Breen et al.[38]	Prospective cohort	589	453	1–2 months
Patel et al.[43]	Prospective cohort	242	53	6 months
Russell et al.[40]	Prospective cohort	319	131	3 months
Macarthur et al.[35]	Prospective cohort	164	165	6 weeks
Macarthur et al.[39]	Prospective cohort	121	123	1 year
Breen et al.[42]	Randomised controlled trial	120	52	6–8 weeks
Howell et al.[8]	Randomised controlled trial	162 166	151 158	3 months 1 year
Thompson et al.[41]	Prospective cohort	433	850	8 weeks 16 weeks 24 weeks
Loughnan et al.[37]	Randomised controlled trial	249	259	6 months

back pain they had one day post partum. When asked about back pain at six weeks post partum, only 12·5% could accurately recall previously reported pain.[34] Retrospective studies were also of limited reliability because the incidence of pre-existing back pain, a known predictor of post-partum back pain, was not balanced. For these reasons, this analysis is restricted to randomised controlled trials and prospective studies that attempted to balance important pre-pregnancy demographics.

To date, there have been two published randomised controlled trials and five prospective cohort studies that have compared the incidence of post-partum back pain in patients who received epidural analgesia and those that did not.[35–41] Two additional studies are available in abstract form.[42,43] Each of the studies identified long-term back pain as an a-priori outcome of the study, and each had at least a 70% follow-up rate. The follow-up period was between four weeks and one year. Some of the studies reported the outcome at several time points. The characteristics of these studies are shown in Table 6.2. In total, 2278 patients received epidural analgesia (or combined spinal–epidural analgesia) and 2114 did not. None of the studies found a statistically significant difference in the incidence of post-partum back pain between groups (Figure 6.4a). None of the studies that used logistic

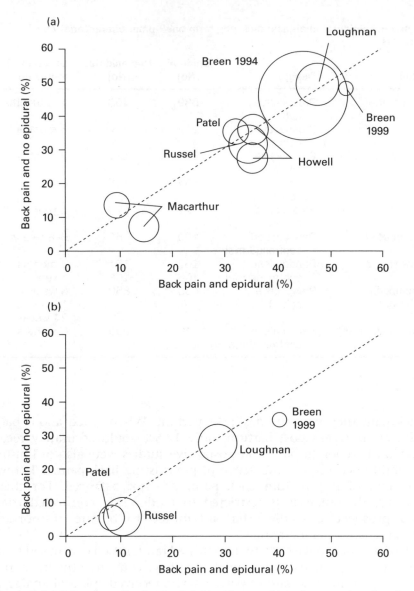

Figure 6.4 (a) Event scatter for the total incidence of long-term post-partum back pain. (b) Event scatter for the incidence of new onset post-partum back pain. In both graphs the size of the circle is proportional to the size of the study

regression found that epidural analgesia was a significant predictor of post-partum low back pain.

The incidence of back pain in the general population is high, and pre-existing back pain is one of the most significant predictors of post-partum back pain.[38] Four of the studies[37,38,40,43] reported the incidence of new onset of post-partum back pain. The incidence was strikingly similar between the two groups (Figure 6.4b). We can therefore conclude that there is no causal association between the use of epidural analgesia and long-term post-partum back pain. This is also true for new onset back pain. This conclusion agrees with a recent systematic review, although the criteria for study inclusion were different.[44]

Ropivacaine versus bupivacaine for labour analgesia

Epidural bupivacaine has been used for many years for labour analgesia. Although this agent has provided excellent sensory analgesia, some patients experienced unacceptable motor block when high concentrations were used. Ropivacaine was developed to reduce these side effects and was released for clinical use in 1996. Since that time, there have been numerous studies performed to determine whether or not ropivacaine was suitable for labour analgesia and whether or not the agent was superior to bupivacaine.

In 1998, a meta-analysis of selected randomised trials concluded that there was an increased rate of spontaneous vaginal delivery with a concomitant reduction in forceps delivery rate in patients who received ropivacaine compared with bupivacaine. The authors also noted better neonatal outcomes as measured by the neuroadaptive capacity score (NACS) in babies exposed to ropivacaine.[45]

Since that time there have been numerous publications comparing the two drugs. Importantly, many studies used low concentrations of both drugs, making their findings more applicable to today's Obstetrical Anaesthesia practice. To date, there have been 27 randomised controlled trials, written in English, that compared epidural bupivacaine to ropivacaine for labour analgesia. A recent meta-analysis[46] included 23 of these[47-69] and an additional four have been published.[70-73] In these studies, 1236 parturients received bupivacaine and 1223 received ropivacaine.

Table 6.3 shows the results when all the studies are combined. There was no difference between any of the outcomes measured except for motor block. The significant heterogeneity between studies for this outcome may be accounted for clinically by the different ways in which the drugs were administered (patient-controlled, continuous infusion, and by clinician top-up), different concentrations of the drugs, and some differences in the timing of the measurement after the local anaesthetic was given. In most cases, motor block was mild and therefore the clinical importance is difficult to determine. The largest clinical trial[56] showed a difference in motor block only after six hours (Figure 6.5).

There is some evidence to suggest that ropivacaine is less potent than bupivacaine.[74,75] This may account for the decrease in motor

Table 6.3 Ropivacaine vs bupivacaine: obstetrical, neonatal and anaesthetic outcomes

Outcome	No of studies included	Bupivacaine n/N or N	Ropivacaine n/N or N	OR or WMD (95% CI)	P value
Obstetrical outcomes					
Spontaneous vaginal delivery	24	606/1075	664/1087	1·13 (0·92 to 1·38)	NS
Instrumental delivery	23	279/1054	270/1061	0·90 (0·65 to 1·26)	NS
Caesarean section	23	161/1065	145/1078	0·86 (0·67 to 1·10)	NS
Neonatal outcomes					
Apgar score at 1 minute <7	11	96/735	91/744	0·92 (0·67 to 1·27)	NS
Apgar score at 5 minutes <7	7	15/791	16/799	0·99 (0·49 to 2·02)	NS
Anaesthetic outcomes					
Time to block onset (minutes)	12	506	513	0·79 (−0·4 to 2·0)	NS
Inadequate analgesia	8	27/337	23/336	0·71 (0·37 to 1·36)	NS
No motor block	27	675/1130	783/1155	1·71 (1·16 to 2·5)	0·007
Maternal satisfaction (VAS score in mm, 0 to 100)	4	443	438	−1·24 (−5·21 to 2·73)	NS

CI = confidence interval; OR = odds ratio; VAS = visual analogue scale; WMD = weighted mean difference

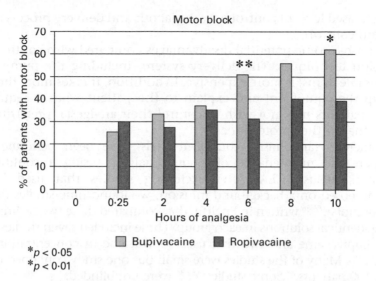

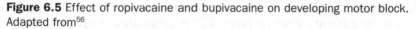

Figure 6.5 Effect of ropivacaine and bupivacaine on developing motor block. Adapted from[56]

block seen with ropivacaine. It should be noted that 21 of the 27 trials compared equal concentrations of bupivacaine with ropivacaine. Whether or not the reduction in motor block is due to differences in potency or to intrinsic properties of the drugs cannot be determined from the current data.

Patient-controlled epidural analgesia versus continuous infusion for labour analgesia

The presence of an epidural catheter enables the clinician to maintain analgesia throughout the first and second stages of labour. Since the 1980s, the parturient has often been given a low dose of local anaesthetic, with or without an opioid such as fentanyl or sufentanil, as a continuous infusion. This avoids several problems associated with clinician-administered intermittent bolus techniques, such as uneven analgesia and potential local anaesthetic toxicity. However, many patients still required local anaesthetic boluses from the clinician, and some had an unacceptably dense motor block of the lower extremities.

In 1988, Gambling *et al.* described patient-controlled epidural analgesia (PCEA) for labour pain. This technique enabled the patient to match the dose of analgesia to the pain as the labour progressed. It also allowed for patient variability in dose requirements. Finally, patient satisfaction may be increased by allowing the patient to have an increased level of control over the labour and delivery process (that is, pain control).[76]

PCEA has some potential disadvantages compared with continuous infusion techniques. The delivery system, including the pump and disposable items, is more expensive. In addition, it takes more time to set up the equipment and explain to the patient what is required. Some patients may not wish to control their analgesia, preferring to leave that to the "professionals".

Numerous randomised controlled trials have been performed to compare the maintenance of labour analgesia using a continuous infusion versus PCEA. After excluding studies that used PCEA superimposed on a background infusion, we found nine studies (in 10 manuscripts),[77–86] written in English, that compared these two techniques using identical solutions in each group. These included seven studies that used bupivacaine and two that used ropivacaine in concentrations of 0·1–0·2%. Many of the studies were small but one study contained more than 100 patients.[83] Some studies[78,83,86] were not blinded.

There was a significant decrease in the requirement for top-ups by clinicians in patients who received PCEA compared with those who received a continuous infusion. In addition, patients received more local anaesthetic in the continuous infusion group. This resulted in an increased incidence of maternal motor block. There were no differences in obstetrical or neonatal outcomes, nor were there consistent differences in maternal pain relief or satisfaction (Table 6.4).

PCEA is therefore an important advance in the maintenance of epidural analgesia for labour pain. This modality proved to be as safe for the mother and baby as continuous infusion, and it has several clear benefits. There is a tangible reduction in workload for clinicians by reducing the number of top-ups requested by the patient. A reduction in the number of top-ups also means that the sterile system is broken less frequently, potentially leading to a lower risk of infection or inadvertent administration of the wrong drug. Furthermore, a reduction in the dose of local anaesthetic leads to a reduction in the incidence of maternal motor block. Unfortunately, PCEA did not improve obstetrical outcome. Maternal satisfaction with both methods of administration was high and not different between the groups, perhaps reflecting the fact that there is no good instrument to measure satisfaction and that few patients were enrolled in studies that reported this outcome. More information is needed before PCEA can be recommended to improve maternal satisfaction.

Summary

Over the past 25 years there have been numerous innovations in the initiation and maintenance of epidural analgesia for labour. There is

Table 6.4 PCEA vs continuous infusion. Anaesthetic, obstetric and neonatal outcomes

Outcome	No of Studies	PCEA N (or n/N)	CEI N (or n/N)	WMD or RD (95% CI)	P value
Mean dose of local anesthetic mg/h	7	257	221	WMD −3·92 (−5·38, −2·42)	<0·00001
Motor block: number of patients with no motor weakness	4	151/167	103/129	RD 18% (6%, 31%)	0·003
Maternal satisfaction – VAS scores	4	36/999	144	WMD 3·9 (−2·2, 9·9)	NS
Pain relief: global pain assessment (VAS)	1	30	30	WMD −7·2 (−19·3, 4·8)	NS
Pain relief: pain of labour first stage (VAS)	1	40	44	WMD 3·0 (−0·80, 6·80)	NS
Pain relief: excellent analgesia first stage	1	47/75	54/84	RD 2% (−17%, 13%)	NS
Pain relief: no episodes of distressing pain in first stage	1	55/75	48/84	RD 16% (2%, 31%)	0·03
Pain relief: complete or good analgesia second stage	2	62/95	62/104	RD 5% (−8%, 18%)	NS
Pain relief: pain assessment second stage (VAS)	1	41	44	WMD 20·0 (7·4, 32·6)	0·02
Mode of delivery: caesarean section	9	41/333	51/307	RD 4% (−8%, 1%)	NS
Mode of delivery: instrumental deliveries	9	109/333	98/307	RD 1% (−6%, 8%)	NS

(Continued)

Table 6.4 (Continued)

Outcome	No of Studies	PCEA N (or n/N)	CEI N (or n/N)	WMD or RD (95% CI)	P value
Low Apgar score at 5 minutes	6	4/201	1/164	WMD 0·01 (−0·02, 0·05)	NS
Low Aphgar score at 1 minute	6	23/201	12/164	WMD 0·00 (−0·07, 0·07)	NS
Hypotension	6	4/275	7/246	RD −1% (−3%, 2%)	NS
High sensory block	3	9/153	8/164	RD 1% (−5%, 6%)	NS

CEI = continuous epidural infusion; CI = confidence interval; PCEA = patient-controlled epidural analgesia; RD = risk difference; VAS = visual analogue scale; WMD = weighed mean difference good evidence to suggest that epidural analgesia has no effect on the caesarean section rate, although it may increase the incidence of operative vaginal delivery. By using the lowest possible concentration of local anaesthetic, the latter effect can be reduced. Combined spinal–epidural techniques may have a role to play in reducing initial local anaesthetic requirements, but the effect of this technique on the delivery mode appears to be identical to that of low-dose epidural analgesia. Epidural analgesia provides better analgesia, superior maternal satisfaction with analgesia, and better early neonatal outcome when compared with parenteral opioids. There is an increased incidence of maternal fever with epidural analgesia. The etiology and clinical significance of this finding are currently controversial.

There is good evidence to suggest that epidural analgesia does not cause long-term back pain. This was consistently shown in randomised controlled trials and cohort studies that had high follow-up rates for up to one year.

The role of ropivacaine for labour analgesia is still unclear. There does not appear to be consistent benefit of ropivacaine when compared with bupivacaine when both are used in low concentrations. Some patients may benefit from the use of ropivacaine because of the reduction of motor block after prolonged (six hours or more) use.

PCEA may be beneficial for the maintenance of labour analgesia. Compared with continuous infusion, it may take more time to set up the equipment and educate the patient. In addition, there are some patients who may not wish (or be able) to participate in its use. However, PCEA reduces the amount of local anaesthetic and motor block in parturients. This modality also reduces the need for clinician-initiated top-ups, resulting in reduced workload and the potential for better maintenance of sterility at the epidural site. Whether a continuous background infusion superimposed on PCEA provides additional benefit is not yet known.

References

1. Morton SC, Williams MS, Keeler EB, Gambone JC, Kahn KL. Effect of epidural analgesia for labor on the cesarean delivery rate. *Obstet Gynecol* 1994;**83**:1045–52.
2. Lieberman E, Lang JM, Cohen A, D'Agostino RJ, Datta S, Frigoletto FD, Jr. Association of epidural analgesia with cesarean delivery in nulliparas. *Obst Gynecol* 1996;**88**:993–1000.
3. Goldberg AB, Cohen BA, Lieberman E. Nulliparas' preferences for epidural analgesia: their effects on actual use in labor. *Birth* 1999;**26**:139–43.
4. Hess PE, Pratt SD, Soni AK, Sarna MC, Oriol NE. An association between severe labor pain and cesarean delivery. *Anesth Analg* 2000;**90**:881–6.
5. Wuitchik M, Bakal D, Lipshitz J. The clinical significance of pain and cognitive activity in latent labor. *Obstet Gynecol* 1989;**73**:35–42.
6. Bofill JA, Vincent RD, Ross EL. Nulliparous active labor, epidural analgesia, and cesarean delivery for dystocia. *Am J Obstet Gynecol* 1997;**177**:1465–70.

7. Clark A, Carr D, Loyd G, Cook V, Spinnato J. The influence of epidural analgesia on cesarean delivery rates: a randomised, prospective clinical trial. *Am J Obstet Gynecol* 1998;**179**:1527–33.
8. Howell CJ, Kidd C, Roberts W, *et al.* A randomised controlled trial of epidural compared with non-epidural analgesia in labour. *Br J Obstet Gynecol* 2001;**108**:27–33.
9. Loughnan BA, Carli F, Romney M, Doré CJ, Gordon H. Randomised controlled comparison of epidural bupivacaine versus pethidine for analgesia in labour. *Br J Anaesth* 2000;**84**:715–9.
10. Muir HA, Shukla R, Liston R, Writer D. Randomised trial of labour analgesia: a pilot study to compare patient-controlled intravenous analgesia with patient-controlled epidural analgesia to determine if analgesic method affects delivery outcome. *Can J Anaesth* 1996;**43**:A60.
11. Muir HA, Breen T, Campbell D, Halpern SH, Liston R, Blanchard W. A multi-center study of the effects of analgesia on the progress of labor. *Anesthesiology* 2000;A23.
12. Nikkola EM, Ekblad UU, Kero PO, Alihanka JM, Salonen MAO. Intravenous PCA in labor. *Can J Anaesth* 1997;**44**:1248–55.
13. Philipsen T, Jensen N-H. Epidural block or parenteral pethidine as analgesic in labour; a randomised study concerning progress in labour and instrumental deliveries. *Eur J Obstet Gynecol Reprod Biol* 1989;**30**:27–33.
14. Philipsen T, Jensen N-H. Maternal opinion about analgesia in labour and delivery: a comparison of epidural blockade and intramuscular pethidine. *Eur J Obstet Gynecol Reprod Biol* 1990;**34**:205–10.
15. Ramin SM, Gambling DR, Lucas MJ, Sharma SK, Sidawi JE, Leveno KJ. Randomised trial of epidural versus intravenous analgesia during labor. *Obstet Gynecol* 1995;**86**:783–9.
16. Robinson JO, Rosen M, Evans JM, Revill SI, David H, Rees GA. Maternal opinion about analgesia for labour: a controlled trial between epidural block and intramuscular pethidine. *Anaesthesia* 1980;**35**:1173–81.
17. Sharma SK, Sidawi JE, Ramin SM, Lucas MJ, Leveno KJ, Cunningham FG. Cesarean delivery: a randomised trial of epidural versus patient-controlled meperidine analgesia during labor. *Anesthesiology* 1997;**87**:487–94.
18. Sharma SK, Alexander JM, Messick G, *et al.* Cesarean delivery: a randomised trial of epidural analgesia versus intravenous meperidine analgesia during labor in nulliparous women. *Anesthesiology* 2002;**96**:546–51.
19. Thorp JA, Hu DH, Albin RM, *et al.* The effect of intrapartum epidural analgesia on nulliparous labor: a randomised, controlled, prospective trial. *Am J Obstet Gynecol* 1993;**169**:851–8.
20. Leighton BL, Halpern SH. The effects of epidural analgesia on labor, maternal, and neonatal outcomes: a systematic review. *Am J Obst Gynecol* 2002;**186**:S69–S77.
21. Fogel ST, Shyken JM, Leighton BL, Mormol JS, Smeltzer JS. Epidural labor analgesia and the incidence of cesarean delivery for dystocia. *Anesth Analg* 1998;**87**:119–23.
22. Gribble RK, Meier PR. Effect of epidural analgesia on the primary cesarean rate. *Obstet Gynecol* 1991;**78**:231–4.
23. Johnson S, Rosenfeld JA. The effect of epidural analgesia on the length of labor. *J Fam Practice* 1995;**40**:244–7.
24. Lyon DS, Knuckles G, Whitaker E, Salgado S. The effect of instituting an elective labor epidural program on the operative delivery rate. *Obstet Gynecol* 1997;**90**:135–41.
25. Zhang J, Yancey MK, Klebanoff MA, Schwarz J, Schweitzer D. Does epidural analgesia prolong labor and increase risk of cesarean delivery? A natural experiment. *Am J Obstet Gynecol* 2001;**185**:128–34.
26. Segal S, Su M, Gilbert P. The effect of a rapid change in availability of epidural analgesia on the cesarean delivery rate: a meta-analysis. *Am J of Obstet Gynecol* 2000;**183**:974–8.
27. Collis RE, Davies DWL, Aveling W. Randomised comparison of combined spinal–epidural and standard epidural analgesia in labour. *Lancet* 1995;**345**:1413–6.
28. Comparative Obstetric Mobile Epidural Trial (COMET) study group UK. Effect of low-dose mobile versus traditional epidural techniques on mode of delivery: a randomised trial. *Lancet* 2001;**358**:19–23.

29. James KS, McGrady E, Quasim I, Patrick A. Comparison of epidural bolus administration of 0.25% bupivacaine and 0.1% bupivacaine with 0·0002% fentanyl for analgesia during labour. *Br J Anaesth* 1998;**81**:507–10.
30. Nageotte MP, Larson D, Rumney PJ, Sidhu M, Hollenbach K. Epidural analgesia compared with combined spinal–epidural analgesia during labor in nulliparous women. *N Engl J Med* 1997;**337**:1715–9.
31. Angle P, Halpern S, Morgan A. Effect of low dose mobile versus high dose epidural techniques on the progress of labor: a meta-analysis. *Anesthesiology* 2002;**96** (Suppl. 1):P52.
32. Grove LH. Backache, headache and bladder dysfunction after delivery. *Br J Anaesth* 1973;**45**:1147–9.
33. Macarthur C, Lewis M, Knox EG, Crawford JS. Epidural anaesthesia and long term backache after childbirth. *BMJ* 1990;**301**:9–12.
34. Macarthur C, Macarthur A, Weeks S. Accuracy of recall of back pain after delivery. *BMJ* 1996;**313**:467–8.
35. Macarthur A, Macarthur C, Weeks S. Epidural-anesthesia and low-back-pain after delivery: a prospective cohort study. *BMJ* 1995;**311**:1336–9.
36. Howell CJ, Dean T, Lucking L, Dziedzic K, Jones PW, Johanson RB. Randomised study of long term outcome after epidural versus non-epidural analgesia during labour. *BMJ* 2002;**325**:357–9.
37. Loughnan BA, Carli F, Romney M, Dore CJ, Gordon H. Epidural analgesia and backache: a randomised controlled comparison with intramuscular meperidine for analgesia during labour. *Br J Anaesth* 2002;**89**:466–72.
38. Breen TW, Ransil BJ, Groves PA, Oriol NE. Factors associated with back pain after childbirth. *Anesthesiology* 1994;**81**:29–34.
39. Macarthur AJ, Macarthur C, Weeks SK. Is epidural anesthesia in labor associated with chronic low back pain? A prospective cohort study. *Anesth Analg* 1997;**85**:1066–70.
40. Russell R, Dundas R, Reynolds F. Long term backache after childbirth: prospective search for causative factors. *BMJ* 1996;**312**:1384–8.
41. Thompson JF, Roberts CL, Currie M, Ellwood DA. Prevalance and persistence of health problems after childbirth: associations with parity and method of birth. *Birth* 2002;**29**:83–94.
42. Breen TW, Campbell DC, Halpern SH, Muir HA, Blanchard W. Epidural analgesia and back pain following delivery: a prospective randomised study. *Anesthesiology* 1999;**90**:A7.
43. Patel M, Fernando R, Gill P, Urquart J, Morgan B. A prospective study on long-term backache after childbirth in primigravidae: the effect of ambulatory epidural analgesia during labour. *Int J Obstet Anesth* 1995;**4**:187.
44. Lieberman E, O'Donoghue C. Unintended effects of epidural analgesia during labor: a systematic review. *Am J Obst Gynecol* 2002;**186**:S31–S68.
45. Writer WD, Stienstra R, Eddleston JM, *et al*. Neonatal outcome and mode of delivery after epidural analgesia for labour with ropivacaine and bupivacaine: a prospective meta-analysis. *Br J Anaesth* 1998;**81**:713–7.
46. Halpern SH, Walsh VB. Epidural ropivacaine vs bupivacaine for labor analgesia: a meta-analysis. *Anesth Analg* 2003;**96**:1473–9.
47. Campbell DC, Zwack RM, Crone LA, Yip RW. Ambulatory labor epidural analgesia: bupivacaine versus ropivacaine. *Anesth Analg* 2000;**90**:1384–9.
48. Chua NP, Sia AT, Ocampo CE. Parturient-controlled epidural analgesia during labour: bupivacaine vs. ropivacaine. *Anaesthesia* 2001;**56**:1169–73.
49. Eddleston JM, Holland JJ, Griffin RP, Corbett A, Horsman EL, Reynolds F. A double-blind comparison of 0·25% ropivacaine and 0·25% bupivacaine for extradural analgesia in labour. *Br J Anaesth* 1996;**76**:66–71.
50. Fernandez-Guisasola, Serrano ML, Cobo B, *et al*. A comparison of 0·0625% bupivacaine with fentanyl and 0·1% ropivacaine with fentanyl for continuous epidural labor analgesia. *Anesth Analg* 2001;**92**:1261–5.
51. Finegold H, Mandell G, Ramanathan S. Comparison of ropivacaine 0·1%-fentanyl and bupivacaine 0·125%: fentanyl infusions for epidural labour analgesia. *Can J Anaesth* 2000;**47**:740–5.
52. Fischer C, Blanie P, Jaouen E, Vayssiere C, Kaloul I, Coltat J-C. Ropivacaine, 0·1%, plus sufentanil, 0·5 mug/ml, versus bupivacaine, 0·1%, plus sufentanil, 0·5 mug/ml,

using patient-controlled epidural analgesia for labor: a double-blind comparison. *Anesthesiology* 2000;92:1588–93.

53. Gaiser RR, Venkateswaren P, Cheek TG, *et al.* Comparison of 0·25% ropivacaine and bupivacaine for epidural analgesia for labor and vaginal delivery. *J Clin Anesth* 1997;9:564–8.

54. Gatt S, Crooke D, Lockley S, Anderson A, Armstrong P, Aveline C. A double-blind, randomised parallel investigation into the neurobehavioral status and outcome of infants born to mothers receiving epidural ropivacaine 0·25% and bupivacaine 0·25% for analgesia in labor. *Anesth Intens Care* 1996;24:108–9.

55. Gautier P, De Kock M, Van Steenberge A, Miclot D, Fanard L, Hody JL. A double-blind comparison of 0·125% ropivacaine with sufentanil and 0·125% bupivacaine with sufentanil for epidural labor analgesia. *Anesthesiology* 1999;90:772–8.

56. Halpern SH, Breen TW, Campbell DC, *et al.* A multicentered randomised controlled trial comparing bupivacaine to ropivacaine for labor analgesia. *Anesthesiology* 2003 (in press).

57. Hughes D, Hill D, Fee H. A comparison of bupivacaine-fentanyl with ropivacaine-fentanyl by epidural infusion for labor analgesia. *Anesthesiology* 2000;A1051.

58. Irestedt L, Ekblom A, Olofsson C, Dahlstrom AC, Emanuelsson BM. Pharmacokinetics and clinical effect during continuous epidural infusion with ropivacaine 2·5 mg/ml or bupivacaine 2·5 mg/ml for labour pain relief. *Acta Anaesthesiol Scand* 1998;42:890–6.

59. Kessler BV, Thomas H, Gressler S, Probst S, Vettermann J. PCEA during labor: no difference in pain relief between ropivacain 0·1% and bupivacain 0·125% when sufentanil 0,5ug/ml is added. *Anesthesiology* 2000;A1068.

60. McCrae AF, Jozwiak H, McClure JH. Comparison of ropivacaine and bupivacaine in extradural analgesia for the relief of pain in labour. *Br J Anaesth* 1995;74:261–5.

61. McCrae AF, Westerling P, McClure JH. Pharmacokinetic and clinical study of ropivacaine and bupivacaine in women receiving extradural analgesia in labour. *Br J Anaesth* 1997;79:558–62.

62. Meister GC, D'Angelo R, Owen M, Nelson KE, Gaver R. A comparison of epidural analgesia with 0.125% ropivacaine with fentanyl versus 0·125% bupivacaine with fentanyl during labor. *Anesth Analg* 2000;90:632–7.

63. Merson N. A comparison of motor block between ropivacaine and bupivacaine for continuous labor epidural analgesia. *AANA Journal* 2001;69:54–8.

64. Muir HA, Writer D, Douglas J, Weeks S, Gambling D, Macarthur A. Double-blind comparison of epidural ropivacaine 0·25% and bupivacaine 0·25%, for the relief of childbirth pain. *Can J Anaesth* 1997;44:599–604.

65. Owen MD, Thomas JA, Smith T, Harris LC, D'Angelo R. Ropivacaine 0·075% and bupivacaine 0·075% with fentanyl 2 microg/mL are equivalent for labor epidural analgesia. *Anesth Analg* 2002;94:179–83.

66. Owen MD, D'Angelo R, Gerancher JC, *et al.* 0·125% ropivacaine is similar to 0·125% bupivacaine for labor analgesia using patient-controlled epidural infusion. *Anesth Analg* 1998;86:527–31.

67. Parpaglioni R, Capogna G, Celleno D. A comparison between low-dose ropivacaine and bupivacaine at equianalgesic concentrations for epidural analgesia during the first stage of labor. *Int J Obstet Anesth* 2000;9:83–6.

68. Smiley RM, Kim-Lo SH, Goodman SR, Jackson MA, Landau R. Patient controlled epidural analgesia with 0·625% ropivacaine versus bupivacaine with fentanyl during labor. *Anesthesiology* 2000;A1065.

69. Stienstra R, Jonker TA, Bourdrez P, Kuijpers JC, Van Kleef JW, Lundberg U. Ropivacaine 0·25% versus bupivacaine 0·25% for continuous epidural analgesia in labor: a double-blind comparison. *Anesth Analg* 1995;80:285–9.

70. Asik I, Goktug A, Gulay I, Alkis N, Uysalel A. Comparison of bupivacaine 0·2% and ropivacaine 0·2% combined with fentanyl for epidural analgesia during labour. *Eur J Anaesthesiol* 2002;19:263–70.

71. Clement HJ, Caruso L, Lopez F, *et al.* Epidural analgesia with 0·15% ropivacaine plus sufentanil 0·5 mug ml^{-1} versus 0·10% bupivacaine plus sufentanil 0·5 mug ml^{-1}: a double-blind comparison during labour. *Br J Anaesth* 2002;88:809–13.

72. Hofmann-Kiefer K, Saran K, Brederode A, Bernasconi H, Zwissler B, Schwender D. Ropivacaine 2 mg/mL vs. bupivacaine 1·25 mg/mL with sufentanil using patient-controlled epidural analgesia in labour. *Acta Anaesthesiol Scand* 2002;46:316–21.

73. Pirbudak L, Tuncer S, Kocoglu H, Goksu S, Celik C. Fentanyl added to bupivacaine 0·05% or ropivacaine 0·05% in patient-controlled epidural analgesia in labour. *Eur J Anaesthesiol* 2002;**19**:271–5.
74. Capogna G, Celleno D, Fusco P, Lyons G, Columb M. Relative potencies of bupivacaine and ropivacaine for analgesia in labour. *Br J Anaesth* 1999;**82**:371–3.
75. Polley LS, Columb MO, Naughton NN, Wagner DS, van de Ven CJ. Relative analgesic potencies of ropivacaine and bupivacaine for epidural analgesia in labor: implications for therapeutic indexes. *Anesthesiology* 1999;**90**:944–50.
76. Hodnett ED. Pain and women's satisfaction with the experience of childbirth: a systematic review. *Am J Obst Gynecol* 2002;**186**:S160–S172.
77. Boutros A, Blary S, Bronchard R, Bonnet F. Comparison of intermittent epidural bolus, continuous epidural infusion and patient controlled-epidural analgesia during labor. *Int J Obstet Anesth* 1999;**8**:236–41.
78. Collis RE, Plaat FS, Morgan BM. Comparison of midwife top-ups, continuous infusion and patient-controlled epidural analgesia for maintaining mobility after a low-dose combined spinal–epidural. *Br J Anaesth* 1999;**82**:233–6.
79. Curry PD, Pacsoo C, Heap DG. Patient-controlled epidural analgesia in obstetric anaesthetic practice. *Pain* 1994;**57**:125–7.
80. Ferrante FM, Rosinia FA, Gordon C, Datta S. The role of continuous background infusions in patient-controlled epidural analgesia for labor and delivery. *Anesth Analg* 1994;**79**:80–4.
81. Ferrante FM, Barber MJ, Segal M, Hughes NJ, Datta S. 0·0625% bupivacaine with 0.0002% fentanyl via patient-controlled epidural analgesia for pain of labor and delivery. *Clin J Pain* 1995;**11**:121–6.
82. Gambling DR, Huber CJ, Berkowitz J, *et al.* Patient-controlled epidural analgesia in labour: varying bolus dose and lockout interval. *Can J Anaesth* 1993;**40**:211–7.
83. Purdie J, Reid J, Thorburn J, Asbury AJ. Continuous extradural analgesia: comparison of midwife top-ups, continuous infusions and patient controlled administration. *Br J Anaesth* 1992;**68**:580–4.
84. Sia AT, Chong JL. Epidural 0·2% ropivacaine for labour analgesia: parturient-controlled or continuous infusion? *Anaesth Int Care* 1999;**27**:154–8.
85. Smedvig JP, Soreide E, Gjessing L. Ropivacaine 1 mg/ml, plus fentanyl 2 microg/ml for epidural analgesia during labour: is mode of administration important? *Acta Anaesthesiol Scand* 2001;**45**:595–9.
86. Tan S, Reid J, Thorburn J. Extradural analgesia in labour: complications of three techniques of administration. *Br J Anaesth* 1994;**73**:619–23.

7: Intravenous fluids for resuscitation

PETER T-L CHOI

In 1918, Captain WB Cannon described the use of intravenous (IV) fluid for the prevention of wound shock on the battlefield.[1,2] Since then, IV fluid administration has become an integral part of volume resuscitation and replacement in surgical and critically ill patients. However, the choice of IV fluid, the timing of fluid administration, and the volume of fluid remain vigorously debated topics.

Initial rationale for the use of particular IV fluids was based mainly on pharmacological mechanisms and physiological outcomes. Although important, these end points were insufficient to define clinical practice. The effect of IV fluids on clinical outcomes, such as mortality, would be a more compelling reason on which to base one's choice of IV fluid. Unfortunately, attempts to draw conclusions on clinical outcomes based on randomised controlled trials were hampered by small sample sizes and insufficient power, heterogeneous populations, and differences in fluid regimens between studies, despite more than 50 randomised controlled trials being published over the past 40 years. Thus, conclusions on the effect of different IV fluids on morbidity and mortality, which are more likely to influence clinicians, have not been forthcoming from individual randomised controlled trials.

In an attempt to answer some questions relating to fluid therapy, systematic review and meta-analysis have been used to pool the results from randomised controlled trials. The resultant evidence has provided some answers, changed clinical practice, identified areas requiring further research, and, at times, generated controversy. In this chapter, the evidence from systematic reviews on the choice of IV fluids will be reviewed.

Systematic reviews on fluid resuscitation

To identify relevant systematic reviews on fluid resuscitation, the bibliographic databases Medline (1966 to January 2003), Embase (1980 to December 2002), CINAHL (1982 to January 2003), and the Cochrane

Database of Systematic Reviews (2002, Issue 4) were searched for systematic reviews of randomised controlled trials that compared different IV fluid regimens in surgical or critically ill patients. Additional systematic reviews were sought by citation review. Systematic reviews were included if they compared: isotonic crystalloids versus colloids, isotonic crystalloids versus hypertonic crystalloids, hypertonic crystalloids versus colloids, colloids versus colloids, isotonic crystalloids versus hypertonic crystalloid–colloid mixtures, or hypertonic crystalloids versus hypertonic crystalloid–colloid mixtures.

Twenty-one systematic reviews on fluid therapy were found.[3-22] Seven of them were excluded because they did not compare different types of IV fluids: two reviewed IV fluid loading before spinal anaesthesia for caesarean section,[3,4] one reviewed IV fluid loading before regional analgesia for labour,[5] one reviewed volume expansion for treatment of pre-eclampsia,[6] one reviewed volume expansion for treatment of aneurismal subarachnoid haemorrhage,[7] one reviewed the timing and volume of fluid resuscitation in bleeding trauma patients,[8] and one reviewed fluid therapy for abdominal aortic surgery.[9] The remaining 14 systematic reviews compared different IV fluids with regard to all cause mortality,[10-19,21-23] pulmonary oedema,[13] and postoperative bleeding.[20] Their findings are described in this chapter.

Systematic reviews of crystalloids for fluid resuscitation

Isotonic crystalloids versus colloids

The earliest systematic reviews on fluid resuscitation compared isotonic crystalloids to colloids with regard to all cause mortality.[10-13] In general, none of the four meta-analyses found any statistically significant differences in mortality when results from all randomised controlled trials were pooled, although the point estimates of the effect size all favoured isotonic crystalloids (Table 7.1). In patients undergoing surgery unrelated to trauma, point estimates favoured colloids but these were not statistically significant.[11-13]

Similarly, on the basis of the results from six randomised controlled trials, Choi et al. found no statistically significant differences in pulmonary oedema between isotonic crystalloids and colloids, but in this case, the point estimates favoured colloids (relative risk (RR) 0·84; 95% confidence interval (CI) 0·28–2·45) for all populations, as well as for non-trauma and surgical subgroups (Table 7.1).[13] In trauma patients, point estimates favoured isotonic crystalloids (3·66; 0·59–22·8).[13] None of these differences was statistically significant.

Table 7.1 Meta-analyses of randomised controlled trials comparing isotonic crystalloids with colloids with all cause mortality or pulmonary oedema as an outcome

Reference	Population	No of patients (studies; years)	Effect size (95% CI)*
Mortality			
Velanovich 1989[10]	All critically ill	826 (8; 1977–84)	RD −5·7% (−20·8%, 9·4%)
	Trauma	Not reported	RD −12·3% (−29·2%, 4·6%)
	Non-trauma	Not reported	RD 7·8% (−3·4%, 19·0%)
Bisonni et al. 1991[11]	All critically ill	354 (7; 1978–84)	Crystalloid 13·4%; colloid 21·2%
	Abdominal aortic surgery	53 (2; 1979)	Crystalloid 9·6%; colloid 4·5%
	Hypovolaemia	255 (4; 1978–83)	Crystalloid 7·3%; colloid 17·8%
	Pulmonary failure	46 (1; 1984)	Crystalloid 50·0%; colloid 60·0%
Schierhout et al. 1998[12]	All critically ill	1315 (19; 1966–96)	RR 1·19 (0·98, 1·45)
	Trauma	636 (6; 1977–93)	RR 1·30 (0·95, 1·77)
	Surgery	191 (7; 1979–96)	RR 0·55 (0·18, 1·65)
	Burns	416 (4; 1966–83)	RR 1·21 (0·88, 1·66)
Choi et al. 1999[13]†	All critically ill	732 (15; 1977–94)	RR 1·16 (0·86, 1·59)
	Trauma	302 (5; 1977–83)	RR 2·57 (1·12, 5·88)
	Non-trauma	430 (10; 1979–94)	RR 1·02 (0·73, 1·43)
	Surgery	296 (7; 1979–92)	RR 0·94 (0·30, 2·95)
Pulmonary oedema			
Choi et al. 1999[13]†	All critically ill	180 (6; 1979–90)	RR 0·84 (0·28, 2·45)
	Trauma	86 (2; 1981–83)	RR 3·66 (0·59, 22·8)
	Non-trauma	94 (4; 1979–90)	RR 0·47 (0·19, 1·19)
	Surgery	68 (3; 1979–90)	RR 0·74 (0·26, 2·07)

CI = confidence interval; RD = risk difference; RR = relative risk

*For risk differences, RD < 0% favours the crystalloid group; RD > 0% favours the colloid group. For relative risks, RR < 1 favours the colloid group; RR > 1 favours the crystalloid group. Results are statistically significant (P < 0·05) if the 95% CI do not include 0 for risk differences or 1 for relative risks

†Effect sizes and 95% CI have been recalculated as the original calculations in this meta-analysis used RR < 1 to favour the crystalloid group and RR > 1 to favour the colloid group

Hypertonic crystalloids versus isotonic crystalloids

Bunn *et al.* identified 12 randomised controlled trials that compared hypertonic crystalloids to isotonic crystalloids with regard to all cause mortality.[14] Five trials studied 425 trauma patients, three studied 89 burn patients, and four studied 158 surgical patients. No statistically significant differences in mortality were seen. The point estimates favoured hypertonic crystalloids in trauma (0·84; 0·61–1·16) and surgery (0·62; 0·08–4·57) and favoured isotonic crystalloids in burns (1·49; 0·56–3·95).

Hypertonic crystalloids versus colloids

Alderson *et al.* identified three randomised controlled trials that compared hypertonic crystalloids with colloids (albumin, hydroxyethylstarch, and gelatin).[15] Only one trial with 38 patients reported any deaths: three patients died in the albumin group; none died in the hypertonic saline group.[24] The differences were not statistically significant (7·00; 0·39–126·9).

Systematic reviews of specific colloids for fluid resuscitation

Meta-analyses that compare crystalloids with colloids[10-13] have been criticised for pooling heterogeneous classes of colloids. To address this criticism, recent systematic reviews have examined classes of colloids separately. In general, colloids have been classified into human albumin or plasma protein fraction (hereafter abbreviated as "albumin"), starches (mainly hydroxyethylstarch), dextrans, and gelatins.

Albumin or plasma protein fraction

Of all intravenous fluids, albumin has received the most attention, with over 50 randomised controlled trials published as of December 2000. Six meta-analyses have reviewed the evidence from randomised controlled trials of albumin use in fluid resuscitation with regard to all cause mortality[15-19] or postoperative bleeding.[20] The first systematic review on albumin was published concurrently in the *British Medical Journal*[16] and the *Cochrane Database of Systematic Review*. The Cochrane review was subsequently updated.[18] Three systematic reviews compared albumin with crystalloids;[15,17,18] two compared albumin with other colloids.[19,20] Table 7.2 summarises the evidence on albumin.

Wilkes and Navickis identified 42 randomised controlled trials that compared albumin with isotonic or hypertonic crystalloids with no albumin or lower doses of albumin with regard to all cause

Table 7.2 Meta-analyses of randomised controlled trials comparing albumin or plasma protein fraction with crystalloids or other colloids with all cause mortality or postoperative bleeding as an outcome

Reference	Control group	Population	No of patients (studies; years)	Effect size (95% CI)*
Mortality				
Wilkes et al. 2001[17]	Crystalloids with no or lower albumin dose	All patients	2958 (42; 1962–2000)	RR 1·11 (0·95, 1·28)
		Surgery or trauma	1339 (20; 1977–2000)	RR 1·12 (0·85, 1·46)
		Burns	197 (4; 1975–95)	RR 1·76 (0·97, 3·17)
		Hypoalbuminaemia	357 (4; 1988–97)	RR 1·59 (0·91, 2·78)
		High-risk neonates	304 (6; 1973–99)	RR 1·19 (0·78, 1·81)
		Ascites	373 (4; 1962–99)	RR 0·93 (0·67, 1·28)
Alderson et al. 2002[15]	Isotonic crystalloids	All critically ill	641 (18; 1977–97)	RR 1·52 (1·08, 2·13)
Alderson et al. 2002[18]	Isotonic crystalloids or no albumin	All critically ill	1519 (31; 1973–97)	RR 1·52 (1·17, 1·99)
		Hypovolemia	719 (18; 1977–97)	RR 1·46 (0·97, 2·22)
		Burns	163 (3; 1978–95)	RR 2·40 (1·11, 5·19)
		Hypoalbuminaemia	637 (10; 1973–97)	RR 1·38 (0·94, 2·03)
Bunn et al. 2002[19]	Hydroxyethylstarch	All critically ill	1029 (20; 1982–98)	RR 1·17 (0·91, 1·50)
Bunn et al. 2002[19]	Gelatin	All critically ill	542 (4; 1987–96)	RR 0·99 (0·69, 1·42)
Postoperative bleeding				
Wilkes et al. 2001[20]	Hydroxyethylstarch	Cardiopulmonary bypass	653 (16; 1982–98)	SMD −0·24 (−0·40, −0·08)

CI = confidence interval; RR = relative risk; SMD = standardised mean difference

*For relative risks, RR < 1 favours the albumin group; RR > 1 favours the control group. For standardised mean differences, SMD < 0 favours the albumin group; SMD > 0 favours the control group. Results are statistically significant (P < 0·05) if the 95% CI do not include 1 for relative risks or 0 for standardised mean differences

mortality.[17] From their meta-analysis, they concluded that there was no statistically significant difference in mortality between the two groups. However, the point estimates for all study populations, with the exception of ascites, favoured the crystalloid group.

By contrast, the Cochrane Injuries Group Albumin Reviewers completed two systematic reviews comparing albumin to crystalloids.[15,18] In their first meta-analysis, Alderson et al. pooled the results from 18 randomised controlled trials that compared albumin with isotonic crystalloids for fluid resuscitation in critically ill patients. They found a statistically significant increase in mortality in the albumin group (RR 1·52; 95% CI 1·08–2·13). These results were confirmed in their second meta-analysis, which pooled results from 31 randomised controlled trials that compared albumin with isotonic crystalloids, no albumin, or lower doses of albumin. The relative risk for mortality remained unchanged and the 95% CI narrowed (1·17–1·99).

Alderson et al. also found one trial that compared albumin-hypertonic crystalloid with isotonic crystalloid.[15] The trial enrolled only 14 patients and did not find any difference in mortality (0·50; 0·06–4·33).[25]

The results of the three meta-analyses have generated much discussion and some controversy. Alderson and colleagues concluded that the "use of human albumin in critically ill patients should be urgently reviewed and that it should not be used outside the context of a rigorously conducted randomised controlled trial".[18] By contrast, Wilkes and Navickis stated that their "findings should allay concerns about the safety of albumin".[17] The discrepancy in conclusions relate, in part, to the differences in selection criteria for the non-albumin comparative group. Wilkes and Navickis included studies with hypertonic crystalloids; Alderson and colleagues did not. In spite of this difference, concerns about the safety of albumin cannot be dismissed. In all three meta-analyses, the point estimates have favoured the non-albumin group. At this time, one can conclude that there is no benefit to mortality with the use of albumin compared with crystalloids in fluid resuscitation. Given the possibility of discrepant results between meta-analyses of small studies (as in this case) and large randomised controlled trials, whether albumin increases mortality or not remains to be determined.

The efficacy of albumin compared with other colloids has been reviewed in two meta-analyses of randomised controlled trials (Table 7.2). Bunn et al. identified 25 studies that compared albumin to hydroxyethylstarch (20 studies), dextrans (three studies), or gelatins (four studies).[19] There was no statistically significant difference between albumin and hydroxyethylstarch with regard to mortality, but the point estimate favoured the latter (1·17; 0·91–1·50).[19] No deaths were observed in the three studies that compared albumin with dextrans. Three of the four studies that compared albumin with gelatins did not find any deaths. In the one study with deaths, albumin was not significantly better than gelatins in reducing mortality in fluid resuscitation, although the point estimate favoured albumin (0·99; 0·69–1·42).[26]

Wilkes *et al.* compared albumin with hydroxyethylstarch with regard to the amount of postoperative bleeding in patients undergoing cardiopulmonary bypass (Table 7.2).[20] They identified 16 randomised controlled trials and found a statistically significant reduction in postoperative bleeding with albumin (standardised mean difference 0·24; 0·40–0·08).[20] The clinical significance is unclear. In adults (14 trials), the pooled mean blood loss was 693 ± 350 ml in the albumin group compared with 789 ± 487 ml in the hydroxyethylstarch group.[20] No differences between the two colloids were seen in terms of the duration of postoperative ventilatory support or intensive care unit stay, although the standardised mean differences favoured the albumin group in both outcomes.[20]

Starches

Aside from the comparisons with albumin, randomised controlled trials have compared hydroxyethylstarch with other intravenous fluids. Table 7.3 summarises the evidence from meta-analyses of these trials. Alderson *et al.* identified seven trials that compared hydroxyethylstarch with isotonic crystalloids.[15] No difference in mortality was seen between the two groups but the point estimate favoured isotonic crystalloids (1·16; 0·68–1·96). Bunn *et al.* found 11 trials that compared hydroxyethylstarch with gelatins. Again, there was no difference in mortality (1·00; 0·78–1·28).

Dextrans

Randomised controlled trials of fluid resuscitation with dextrans have used varying concentrations (usually 6%) of dextran 70 or mixtures of 7·5% hypertonic saline with 6% dextran 70 (hypertonic saline–dextran). Table 7.4 summarises the evidence from meta-analyses of these trials.

Two systematic reviews have compared dextran 70 to isotonic crystalloids with regards to all cause mortality in fluid resuscitation.[15,22] In both meta-analyses, there was no statistically significant difference in mortality between the dextran 70 and isotonic crystalloids (Table 7.4). Point estimates favoured the use of isotonic crystalloids.

Wade and colleagues compared hypertonic saline–dextran with isotonic crystalloids with regard to all cause mortality in fluid resuscitation of trauma patients.[21–23] Two systematic reviews[21,22]

Table 7.3 Meta-analyses of randomised controlled trials comparing hydroxyethylstarch with crystalloids or other colloids with all cause mortality as an outcome*

Reference	Control group	Population	No of patients (studies; years)	Effect size (95% CI)*
Alderson et al. 2002[15]	Isotonic crystalloids	All critically ill	197 (7; 1983–99)	RR 1·16 (0·68, 1·96)
Bunn et al. 2002[19]	Gelatin	All critically ill	945 (11; 1994–2001)	RR 1·00 (0·78, 1·28)

CI = confidence interval; RR = relative risk

*Comparisons of hydroxyethylstarch to albumin or plasma protein fraction are shown in Table 7.2

†For relative risks, RR < 1 favours the hydroxyethylstarch group; RR > 1 favours the control group. Results are statistically significant (p < 0·05) if the 95% CI do not include 1 for relative risks

Table 7.4 Meta-analyses of randomised controlled trials comparing 6% dextran 70 or 7·5% saline/6% dextran 70 with isotonic crystalloids with all cause mortality as an outcome*

Reference	Population	No of patients (studies; years)	Effect size (95% CI)*
6% dextran 70 Wade et al.[22†]	Traumatic hypotension	719 (5; 1988–93)	OR 1·02 (0·74, 1·40)
Alderson et al.[15]	All critically ill	668 (8; 1978–95)	RR 1·24 (0·94, 1·65)
7.5% saline/6% dextran 70 Wade et al.[21†]	Traumatic hypotension	Unclear (8; 1989–94)	OR 0·68 (0·48, 0·96)
Wade et al.[22†]	Traumatic hypotension	1233 (8; 1989–94)	OR 0·83 (0·64, 1·06)
Wade et al.[23†]	Traumatic brain injury	223 (6; 1990–3)	OR 0·47 (0·22, 0·99)

CI = confidence interval; OR = odds ratio; RR = relative risk
*For odds ratios and relative risks, OR < 1 and RR < 1 favour the dextran group; OR > 1 and RR > 1 favour the crystalloid group. Results are statistically significant (P < 0·05) if the 95% CI do not include 1
†Effect sizes and 95% CI have been recalculated as the original calculations in this meta-analysis used OR < 1 to favour the crystalloid group and OR > 1 to favour the dextran group

examined the same studies, although one used meta-analysis of individual patient data[21] and the other did not.[22] The former reported a statistically significant reduction in mortality with hypertonic saline–dextran in the treatment of traumatic hypotension; the latter found no difference, although the point estimate favoured the hypertonic saline–dextran group (Table 7.4). The third systematic review also used meta-analysis of individual patient data and reported a statistically significant reduction in mortality with hypertonic saline–dextran in the treatment of traumatic brain injury (Table 7.4).[23]

Bunn et al. identified two randomised controlled trials that compared dextran 70 with gelatin in fluid resuscitation.[19] There were only 42 patients in total and no deaths were observed in both studies.

Gelatins

Alderson et al. identified four randomised controlled trials with 95 patients that compared gelatins with isotonic crystalloids with regard to all cause mortality in critically ill patients. There was no statistically significant difference in mortality between the two groups, although the point estimate favoured the gelatin group (0·50; 0·08–3·03).

Summary of the current evidence

On the basis of meta-analyses of randomised controlled trials, the use of albumin, hydroxyethylstarch, or dextrans does not reduce mortality compared with isotonic crystalloids in the resuscitation of critically ill patients. Hypertonic crystalloids or hypertonic crystalloid–dextran solutions may reduce mortality compared with isotonic crystalloids in the resuscitation of trauma patients. Whether one colloid is better or worse than another colloid is still controversial. Hydroxyethylstarch may be better than albumin with regard to mortality in critically ill patients; however, postoperative bleeding after coronary artery bypass surgery is lower with albumin compared with hydroxyethylstarch. There may be fewer episodes of pulmonary oedema with the use of colloids compared with isotonic crystalloids.

Limitations to the current evidence

Although the meta-analyses in this chapter represent the best evidence regarding choice of intravenous fluid for resuscitation, one should be cautious in the application of their findings. Firstly, all of the meta-analyses pooled results from small randomised controlled trials. Most trials enrolled fewer than 100 patients per group. Most of the meta-analyses had fewer than 200 outcome events per comparison, which would be considered "small" and should be interpreted with caution.[27] Previous instances, such as magnesium in the treatment of acute myocardial infarction and hormone replacement therapy in the prevention of coronary artery disease, in which subsequent large randomised controlled trials have contradicted the results of meta-analyses of small trials, highlight the danger of overinterpreting the findings of these systematic reviews.

Secondly, although most of the systematic reviews have attempted to address sources of heterogeneity such as methodological issues, types of colloids, and patient populations, the fluid regimens and co-interventions varied between individual clinical trials. A glance at the span of years over which these trials were published suggests that some of the fluid regimens may be outdated. Pooling of such trials may be inappropriate.

Thirdly, aside from mortality, other clinical outcomes, such as pulmonary oedema, acute renal failure, neurological sequelae, and coagulopathy, have not been studied sufficiently. Also, data on adverse events, including prion-related diseases with the use of human-derived (albumin or plasma protein fraction) or animal-derived (gelatins) products and allergic reactions, are still rare. The effect of an intravenous fluid on these outcomes and adverse events can influence one's choice of fluid.

The future

The results from the systematic reviews indicate that further research is needed to determine optimal fluid regimens for specific patient populations. Large, adequately powered, well designed, multicentre, randomised controlled trials comparing the effects of modern fluid resuscitation protocols on clinically relevant outcomes are needed. As noted in one recent editorial,[28] at least two such trials are under way. One trial is comparing 4% albumin to 0·9% saline with regards to 28-day mortality in critically ill patients and is powered to detect a 3% difference. A second trial is comparing hypertonic saline to isotonic crystalloid in patients with hypotensive traumatic brain injury with regard to neurological sequelae. Hopefully, additional trials will be under way in the future.

References

1. Cannon WB. Acidosis in cases of shock, hemorrhage and gas infection. *JAMA* 1918;**70**:531.
2. Cannon WB, Fraser J, Cowell EM. The preventive treatment of wound shock. *JAMA* 1918;**70**:618–21.
3. Morgan PJ, Halpern SH, Tarshis J. The effects of an increase in central blood volume before spinal anesthesia for cesarean delivery: a qualitative systematic review. *Anesth Analg* 2001;**92**:997–1005.
4. Emmett RS, Cyna AM, Andrew M, Simmons SW. Techniques for preventing hypotension during spinal anaesthesia for caesarean section (Cochrane review). *Cochrane Database Syst Rev* 2002;**4**:CD002251.
5. Hofmeyr GJ. Prophylactic intravenous preloading for regional analgesia in labour (Cochrane review). *Cochrane Database Syst Rev* 2002;**4**:CD000175.
6. Duley L, Williams J, Henderson-Smart DJ. Plasma volume expansion for treatment of pre-eclampsia (Cochrane review). *Cochrane Database Syst Rev* 2002;**4**:CD001805.
7. Feigin VL, Rinkel GJE, Algra A, van Gijn J. Circulatory volume expansion for aneurysmal subarachnoid hemorrhage (Cochrane review). *Cochrane Database Syst Rev* 2002;**4**:CD000483.
8. Kwan I, Bunn F, Roberts I, on behalf of the WHO Pre-Hospital Trauma Care Steering Committee. Timing and volume of fluid administration for patients with bleeding following trauma (Cochrane review). *Cochrane Database Syst Rev* 2002;**4**:CD002245.
9. Whatling PJ. Intravenous fluids for abdominal aortic surgery (Cochrane review). *Cochrane Database Syst Rev* 2002;**4**:CD000991.
10. Velanovich V. Crystalloid versus colloid fluid resuscitation: a meta-analysis of mortality. *Surgery* 1989;**105**:65–71.
11. Bisonni RS, Holtgrave DR, Lawler F, Marley DS. Colloids versus crystalloids in fluid resuscitation: an analysis of randomized controlled trials. *J Fam Pract* 1991;**32**: 387–90.

12. Schierhout G, Roberts I. Fluid resuscitation with colloid or crystalloid solutions in critically ill patients: a systematic review of randomised trials. *BMJ* 1998;**316**:961–4.
13. Choi PT, Yip G, Quinonez LG, Cook DJ. Crystalloids vs. colloids in fluid resuscitation: a systematic review. *Crit Care Med* 1999;**27**:200–10.
14. Bunn F, Roberts I, Tasker R, Akpa E. Hypertonic versus isotonic crystalloid for fluid resuscitation in critically ill patients (Cochrane review). *Cochrane Database Syst Rev* 2002;**4**:CD002045.
15. Alderson P, Schierhout G, Roberts I, Bunn F. Colloids versus crystalloids for fluid resuscitation in critically ill patients (Cochrane review). *Cochrane Database Syst Rev* 2002;**4**:CD000567.
16. Human albumin administration in critically ill patients: systematic review of randomised controlled trials. Cochrane Injuries Group Albumin Reviewers. *BMJ* 1998;**317**:235–40.
17. Wilkes MM, Navickis RJ. Patient survival after human albumin administration: a meta-analysis of randomized, controlled trials. *Ann Intern Med* 2001;**135**:149–64.
18. Alderson P, Bunn F, Lefebvre C, *et al.* Human albumin solution for resuscitation and volume expansion in critically ill patients (Cochrane review). *Cochrane Database Syst Rev* 2002;**4**:CD001208.
19. Bunn F, Alderson P, Hawkins V. Colloid solutions for fluid resuscitation (Cochrane review). *Cochrane Database Syst Rev* 2002;**4**:CD001319.
20. Wilkes MM, Navickis RJ, Sibbald WJ. Albumin versus hydroxyethyl starch in cardiopulmonary bypass surgery: a meta-analysis of postoperative bleeding. *Ann Thorac Surg* 2001;**72**:527–34.
21. Wade C, Grady J, Kramer G. Efficacy of hypertonic saline dextran (HSD) in patients with traumatic hypotension: a meta-analysis of individual patient data. *Acta Anaesthesiol Scand Suppl* 1997;**110**:77–9.
22. Wade CE, Kramer GC, Grady JJ, Fabian TC, Younes RN. Efficacy of hypertonic 7·5% saline and 6% dextran-70 in treating trauma: a meta-analysis of controlled clinical studies. *Surgery* 1997;**122**:609–16.
23. Wade CE, Grady JJ, Kramer GC, Younes RN, Gehlsen K, Holcroft JW. Individual patient cohort analysis of the efficacy of hypertonic saline/dextran in patients with traumatic brain injury and hypotension. *J Trauma* 1997;**42**:S61–5.
24. Bowser-Wallace BH, Caldwell FT jr. A prospective analysis of hypertonic lactated saline v. Ringer's lactate-colloid for the resuscitation of severely burned children. *Burns* 1986;**12**:402–9.
25. Jelenko C, 3rd. Fluid therapy and the HALFD method. *J Trauma* 1979;**19(11 Suppl)**:866–7.
26. Stockwell MA, Scott A, Day A, Riley B, Soni N. Colloid solutions in the critically ill. A randomised comparison of albumin and polygeline: 2. Serum albumin concentration and incidences of pulmonary oedema. *Anaesthesia* 1992;**47**:7–9.
27. Flather MD, Farkouh ME, Pogue JM, Yusuf S. Strengths and limitations of meta-analysis: larger studies may be more reliable. *Controlled Clin Trials* 1997;**18**:568–79.
28. Cook D, Guyatt G. Colloid use for fluid resuscitation: evidence and spin. *Ann Intern Med* 2001;**135**:205–8.

8: Postoperative nausea and vomiting

MARTIN R TRAMÈR

Postoperative nausea and vomiting (PONV) is a disorder that is frequently underestimated because it is self-limiting, never becomes chronic, and almost never kills. However, there is evidence that 10% of the population have surgery each year,[1] and about 30% of them will develop PONV,[2] which is equal to 2 000 000 people in the United Kingdom alone. Surgical patients prefer postoperative pain to PONV,[3] and would be willing to pay substantial amounts of money for an effective anti-emetic.[4] About 1% of patients who undergo ambulatory surgery are admitted overnight because of uncontrolled PONV.[2] Thus, the economic impact of PONV on healthcare resources may be substantial.

Hundreds of randomised trials on issues related to the control of PONV have been published during the past 40 years. Data from a large number of these trials have been summarised in more than 30 systematic reviews, and this chapter will summarise the results from those. The reviews are about anti-emetics that are used in strabismus surgery;[5] about the usefulness of using propofol,[6,7] or omitting nitrous oxide,[8-10] or avoiding antagonism of neuromuscular blockade;[11] about the anti-emetic efficacy of metoclopramide,[12] droperidol,[13,14] dexamethasone,[15-17] ondansetron,[18-21] tropisetron,[22] dimenhydrinate,[23] or transdermal scopolamine;[24] about the efficacy of anti-emetic interventions that are used to prevent opioid-induced nausea and vomiting;[25,26] about ginger root;[27] and about nonpharmacological techniques that are thought to be anti-emetic (for instance, transcutaneous electrical nerve stimulation).[28]

Some systematic reviews tested the potentially synergistic effect of two anti-emetic drugs – for instance, the combination of a 5-HT$_3$ (5-hydroxytryptamine) receptor antagonist with droperidol,[29] or of a 5-HT$_3$ receptor antagonist with dexamethasone.[15]

Some systematic reviews attempted to establish the relative efficacy of anti-emetic interventions (ondansetron, metoclopramide, and droperidol) through the analysis of direct (head-to-head) comparisons.[30-32]

Finally, an important number of systematic reviews were on methodological issues in PONV trials: the variability in event rates in PONV trials and its implication for estimating the relative efficacy of anti-emetic interventions;[33] the quantitative impact of duplicate publication of PONV trials on the estimation of treatment effect;[34] cost-effectiveness analyses that compare pharmacological strategies to prevent PONV with strategies to treat established symptoms;[35,36] efficacy of anti-emetics in patient groups with different underlying risks (for instance, those with motion sickness or with a history of previous PONV);[37,38] potential ethical problems that may arise from placebo-controlled PONV trials;[39] doubtful validity of PONV data emerging from one single centre;[40] and the problems of direct comparisons in PONV trials without placebo controls.[30]

This large amount of data, systematically searched, critically appraised, and quantitatively summarised, enables an improved understanding of many confusing issues related to the control of PONV and forms the basis for recent advances in the control of PONV. The relative efficacy of many anti-emetic interventions and their potential for harm have been established both for prophylaxis[2] and for the treatment of PONV.[41] Given that systematic reviews tell us what we know and, as a consequence, what we don't know, a rational and thus ethical research agenda has been defined.[42] And finally, an international expert panel has produced clinical guidelines for the control of PONV, taking into account data from these systematic reviews.[43]

This chapter will present a summary of these advances. The rational approach to an improved control of PONV may be structured into six subheadings: identification of patients at risk; keeping the baseline risk low; combination of anti-emetic drugs; prophylaxis is reserved to high-risk patients; abstain from using interventions that have no proven efficacy; and the role of anti-emetics in the control of opioid-related emesis.

Identification of patients at risk

Treatment stratification through the identification of predictive factors for PONV has been the subject of many studies during the past 10 years.[44–48] These studies identified some risk factors that were more likely than others to predict PONV (for instance, female gender, smoking status, opioid use, or a positive history of PONV), and excluded others (for instance, menstrual cycle[49] or an increased body mass index[50]). Laudable attempts to produce scores that may accurately predict PONV in individual patients, and thus help clinicians to target prophylaxis, were shown to have relatively low discriminating power.[51] Also, the definition of some of the predictive factors remained unclear. For instance, for nicotine receptors, there may be a biological basis for their involvement in PONV;[52] it is, however, not known how many cigarettes a day and for how long a period a patient needs to smoke to profit from this "PONV protective" effect. Also, there has been a controversy among authors of different risk factor models, as to whether or not surgery itself was a predictive factor for PONV. The most likely explanation for this uncertainty is that in the various multivariate analyses, nausea and vomiting have not been considered as distinct end points. The most recent risk factor analysis made this distinction at last, and came to the conclusion that some surgeries (for instance, urological, abdominal, or gynaecological interventions) were indeed independent risk factors, but for nausea only, not for vomiting.[53] In conclusion, a risk factor score for PONV should not be regarded as a rule but as a tool for the stratification of patients. Given the relatively low sensitivity and specificity of the various scores that have been proposed, there will always be patients who vomit despite the absence of recognised risk factors, and there will be patients who should actually vomit but don't.

Keeping the baseline risk low

Anaesthetists have no influence on patient-related or surgery-related risk factors for PONV. However, they can adjust the anaesthesia technique if necessary. The simplest way to keep the anaesthesia-related PONV baseline risk low is to avoid general anaesthesia altogether, and to choose a loco-regional anaesthesia technique. This may be a valid option for those who practise loco-regional anaesthesia rarely. When opioids are added to an epidural or spinal anaesthesia, these potentially beneficial and low emetogenic techniques are likely to induce a risk of nausea and vomiting that is comparable to a general anaesthetic.

When anaesthetists choose a general anaesthetic, there are several ways to keep the PONV baseline risk as low as possible: using a propofol anaesthetic (that is, propofol for both induction and maintenance), omitting nitrous oxide, and avoiding the reversal of neuromuscular blockade at the end of surgery. All three techniques decrease the likelihood of PONV to some extent; none, however, is universally effective. Whether the combination of all three further decreases the baseline risk is likely but has never been shown. Avoiding intra-operative opioids may also have a beneficial effect on the PONV baseline risk.[54] However, a "dose–response" of the emetogenic effect of the various opioids and their relative emetogenic potency are not well understood.

Combination of anti-emetic drugs

Most anti-emetic drugs that have been systematically reviewed are efficacious to some extent for preventing PONV: $5-HT_3$ receptor antagonists (for instance, ondansetron or tropisetron), dopamine D_2

receptor antagonists (droperidol), anticholinergics (scopolamine), antihistamines (dimehydrinate), and corticosteroids (dexamethasone). For some drugs, a dose–response curve has been established (ondansetron). For some, the dose–response curve was shown to be almost flat, indicating that very low doses are as effective as much higher doses (droperidol). For yet some others, the original data did not enable the dose–response relation to be established (scopolamine, dimenhydrinate). Some anti-emetics have been shown to have a more pronounced anti-vomiting effect (ondansetron), whereas others have a more prominent anti-nausea effect (droperidol). None of these drugs is universally effective; none can be regarded as the gold standard. The best degree of anti-emetic efficacy that can be expected in high-risk patients (those who would have a PONV rate of 40–80% without prophylaxis) is a number needed to treat (NNT) of about 5 to prevent PONV, compared with a placebo. Thus, at best 20% of high-risk patients who receive a prophylaxis with one of these anti-emetic drugs are likely to profit. Also, all these drugs induce a finite risk of adverse effects. In conclusion, PONV prophylaxis with a single drug may not be regarded as being worthwhile.

As a consequence, these drugs should not be used alone, but should be combined (balanced anti-emesis). The idea of this concept is to profit from an additive or even a synergistic effect of molecules that act at different receptor systems. Ideally, lower doses as with single-drug regimens could be used, and thus the risk of adverse drug reactions could be lowered. For two combinations there is strong evidence from systematic reviews of randomised trials for improved efficacy compared with each drug alone; these are a 5-HT$_3$ receptor antagonist (for instance, ondansetron) combined with droperidol, and a 5-HT$_3$ receptor antagonist combined with dexamethasone. Using a triple association (for instance, a 5-HT$_3$ receptor antagonist plus droperidol plus dexamethasone) seems to be a reasonable strategy to further improve the efficacy of these molecules; this, however, remains to be shown. Dexamethasone should be administered at the beginning of surgery; a 5-HT$_3$ receptor antagonist and droperidol are added at the end. The optimal regimens of these combinations (doses, repeated administrations) and the efficacy of other combinations are unknown.

Prophylaxis is reserved for high-risk patients

Because PONV may be regarded as a minor and self-limiting medical problem that does not become chronic or does not kill, a rational risk–benefit estimation becomes particularly important, especially when patients receive these drugs prophylactically, since not all of these patients actually need the drug. In high-risk patients, a prophylactic multimodal approach should be chosen – that is, an anaesthetic strategy that keeps the baseline risk low, combined with balanced pharmacological anti-emesis. The difficulty then is to define what "high-risk" actually means and to identify these patients accordingly with confidence. In this context, the perception of risk may depend on many factors and on the particular circumstances. For instance, will surgery be performed on an outpatient basis? The patient should then be discharged within hours after surgery. Is the patient a child? The threshold for withholding prophylaxis may be higher in children. The problem in the paediatric setting is that, often, knowledge on efficacy and harm of anti-emetic interventions has to be extrapolated from trials that have been performed in adults. Does the patient have a history of PONV? These patients are often very distressed and apprehensive before surgery. Is there a surgical reason to prevent PONV? A patient with wired jaws, for instance, must not vomit. For patients who do not fall into one of these categories, the "wait-and-see" strategy may be chosen; prophylaxis is avoided and established PONV symptoms are treated as indicated. The advantage of the treatment strategy is that only patients who actually need an anti-emetic will receive it; fewer patients will be exposed to unnecessary adverse drug reactions, and costs may be saved.

The only drug class that has been adequately studied in randomised controlled trials for the treatment of PONV is the group of 5-HT$_3$ receptor antagonists.[41] These trials allow us to draw several important conclusions on the role of 5-HT$_3$ receptor antagonists in the control of PONV. Firstly, despite considerable differences in pharmacokinetics, there is no evidence of any difference in the anti-emetic efficacy between the different 5-HT$_3$ receptor antagonists that have been studied so far. Compared with placebo, single intravenous doses of ondansetron, dolasetron, tropisetron or granisetron have an NNT of 3–4 to prevent further PONV in a nauseous or vomiting patient and up to 24 hours. Secondly, for none of these 5-HT$_3$ receptor antagonists, when used for the treatment of established symptoms, there is evidence of a clinically relevant dose–response relation. Doses that correspond to one quarter to one half of the effective prophylactic doses are good enough for treatment (for instance, ondansetron 1–2 mg, or tropisetron 0·5–1 mg). This, again, may decrease the risk of adverse drug reactions and have an economic impact. Thirdly, 5-HT$_3$ receptor antagonists show consistently a weaker anti-nausea and a stronger anti-vomiting effect. This reinforces the strategy to use combinations of anti-emetic drugs.

Abstain from using interventions that do not have worthwhile efficacy

Anti-emetic interventions should not be used if they have no proven efficacy or if their efficacy is not worthwhile (the NNT to prevent

PONV is, say, above 7). To these interventions belong propofol for induction,[6] metoclopramide,[12] and ginger root.[27] Cannabinoids have shown some efficacy for the control of chemotherapy-related sickness; however, their adverse-effect profile (psychosis, depression, hallucination) precludes widespread clinical use and data from the PONV setting are sparse and do not suggest any usfulness.[55]

A special case: the role of anti-emetics in the control of opioid-related emesis

About 30% of surgical patients who receive an analgesic dose of an opioid postoperatively will have nausea or will vomit, independently of whether the opioid was given by the conventional route (intramuscular or subcutaneous) or by an intravenous patient-controlled analgesia (PCA) device.[56] Opioid-induced sickness is, strictly speaking, not PONV. For single-dose prophylaxis, dexamethasone seems to be the most efficacious anti-emetic.[26] When added to an opioid-PCA device, droperidol was shown to be the most efficacious anti-emetic.[25] In that systematic review, there was a lack of evidence for dose-responsiveness for a wide range of droperidol doses from 1·7 to 17 mg per 100 mg of morphine. In a subsequently conducted large randomised dose-finding study, the anti-emetic efficacy of three droperidol regimens were tested – 0·5 mg, 1·5 mg, and 5 mg of droperidol per 100 mg morphine.[57] The largest dose, 5 mg, was anti-emetic and antipruritic, but there was a high incidence of sedation; 1·5 mg was less anti-emetic, still antipruritic, and there was no sedation. The lowest dose tested, 0·5 mg, was not anti-emetic, not antipruritic, and not sedative. The authors concluded that for an optimal risk–benefit ratio, a droperidol dose between 1·5 and 5 mg should be added to 100 mg of morphine in a PCA pump.

Conclusions

Despite an impressive number of published randomised controlled trials, there is still no "gold standard" anti-emetic intervention in the PONV setting. The efficacy of many older anti-emetic drugs is still poorly understood, and their adverse effect profiles are not well defined. However, the relative efficacy of many anti-emetic interventions has been quantified, both for the prevention of PONV and for the treatment of established symptoms. These drugs should be combined for improved efficacy. Models have been established to facilitate the application of the aggregate results of quantitative systematic reviews to the individual patient level (Chapter 13). More research is needed to further improve dissemination of best evidence practices, and to foster implementation of evidence-based PONV guidelines.

Acknowledgement

Dr Tramèr was supported by a PROSPER grant (No 3233-051939.97/2) from the Swiss National Research Foundation.

References

1. Clergue F, Auroy Y, Pequignot F, Jougla E, Lienhart A, Laxenaire MC. French survey of anesthesia in 1996. *Anesthesiology* 1999;**91**:1509–20.
2. Tramèr MR. A rational approach to the control of postoperative nausea and vomiting: evidence from systematic reviews. Part I. Efficacy and harm of antiemetic interventions, and methodological issues. *Acta Anaesthesiol Scand* 2001;**45**:4–13.
3. VanWijk MGF, Smalhout B. A postoperative analysis of the patient's view of anaesthesia in a Netherlands' teaching hospital. *Anaesthesia* 1990;**45**:679–82.
4. Gan T, Sloan F, Dear G, El-Moalem HE, Lubarsky DA. How much are patients willing to pay to avoid postoperative nausea and vomiting? *Anesth Analg* 2001;**92**:393–400.
5. Tramèr M, Moore A, McQuay H. Prevention of vomiting after paediatric strabismus surgery: a systematic review using the numbers-needed-to-treat method. *Br J Anaesth* 1995;**75**:556–61.
6. Tramèr M, Moore A, McQuay H. Propofol anaesthesia and postoperative nausea and vomiting: quantitative systematic review of randomized controlled studies. *Br J Anaesth* 1997;**78**:247–55.
7. Sneyd JR, Carr A, Byrom WD, Bilski AJT. A meta-analysis of nausea and vomiting following maintenance of anaesthesia with propofol or inhalational agents. *Eur J Anaesthesiol* 1998;**15**:433–45.
8. Tramèr M, Moore A, McQuay H. Omitting nitrous oxide in general anaesthesia: meta-analysis of intraoperative awareness and postoperative emesis in randomized controlled trials. *Br J Anaesth* 1996;**76**:186–93.
9. Divatia J, Vaidya JS, Badwe RA, Hawaldar RW. Omission of nitrous oxide during anesthesia reduces the incidence of postoperative nausea and vomiting: a meta-analysis. *Anesthesiology* 1996;**85**:1055–62.
10. Hartung J. Twenty-four of twenty-seven studies show a greater incidence of emesis associated with nitrous oxide than with alternative anesthetics. *Anesth Analg* 1996;**83**:114–6.
11. Tramèr MR, Fuchs-Buder T. Omitting reversal of neuromuscular blockade: effect on postoperative nausea and vomiting and risk of residual paralysis. A systematic review. *Br J Anaesth* 1999;**82**:379–86.
12. Henzi I, Walder B, Tramèr MR. Metoclopramide in the prevention of postoperative nausea and vomiting: a quantitative systematic review of randomised placebo-controlled studies. *Br J Anaesth* 1999;**83**:761–71.
13. Eberhart LH, Morin AM, Seeling W, Bothner U, Georgieff M. Meta-analysis of controlled randomized studies on droperidol for prevention of postoperative phase vomiting and nausea. *Anasthesiol Intensivmed Notfallmed Schmerzther* 1999;**34**: 528–36.
14. Henzi I, Sonderegger J, Tramèr MR. Efficacy, dose–response, and adverse effects of droperidol for prevention of postoperative nausea and vomiting. *Can J Anesth* 2000;**47**:537–51.
15. Henzi I, Walder B, Tramèr MR. Dexamethasone for the prevention of postoperative nausea and vomiting: a quantitative systematic review. *Anesth Analg* 2000;**90**: 186–94.

16. Eberhart LH, Morin AM, Georgieff M. Dexamethasone for prophylaxis of postoperative nausea and vomiting: a meta-analysis of randomized controlled studies. *Anaesthesist* 2000;**49**:713–20.
17. Steward DL, Welge JA, Myer CM. Do steroids reduce morbidity of tonsillectomy? Meta-analysis of randomized trials. *Laryngoscope* 2001;**111**:1712–8.
18. Tramèr MR, Moore RA, Reynolds DJM, McQuay HJ. A quantitative systematic review of ondansetron in treatment of established postoperative nausea and vomiting. *BMJ* 1997;**314**:1088–92.
19. Tramèr MR, Reynolds DJM, Moore RA, McQuay HJ. Efficacy, dose–response, and safety of ondansetron in prevention of postoperative nausea and vomiting: a quantitative systematic review of randomized placebo-controlled trials. *Anesthesiology* 1997;**87**:1277–89.
20. Figueredo ED, Canosa LG. Ondansetron in the prophylaxis of postoperative vomiting: a meta-analysis. *J Clin Anesth* 1998;**10**:211–21.
21. Cox F. Systematic review of ondansetron for the prevention and treatment of postoperative nausea and vomiting in adults. *Br J Theatre Nurs* 1999;**9**:556–66.
22. Kranke P, Eberhart LH, Apfel CC, Broscheit J, Geldner G, Roewer N. Tropisetron for prevention of postoperative nausea and vomiting: a quantitative systematic review. *Anaesthesist* 2002;**51**:805–14.
23. Kranke P, Morin AM, Roewer N, Eberhart LH. Dimenhydrinate for prophylaxis of postoperative nausea and vomiting: a meta-analysis of randomized controlled trials. *Acta Anaesthesiol Scand* 2002;**46**:238–44.
24. Kranke P, Morin AM, Roewer N, Wulf H, Eberhart LH. The efficacy and safety of transdermal scopolamine for the prevention of postoperative nausea and vomiting: a quantitative systematic review. *Anesth Analg* 2002;**95**:133–43.
25. Tramèr MR, Walder B. Efficacy and adverse effects of prophylactic antiemetics during PCA therapy: a quantitative systematic review. *Anesth Analg* 1999;**88**:1354–61.
26. Hirayama T, Ishii F, Yago K, Ogata H. Evaluation of the effective drugs for the prevention of nausea and vomiting induced by morphine used for postoperative pain: a quantitative systematic review. *Yakugaku Zasshi* 2001;**121**:179–85.
27. Ernst E, Pittler MH. Efficacy of ginger for nausea and vomiting: a systematic review of randomized clinical trials. *Br J Anaesth* 2000;**84**:367–71.
28. Lee A, Done ML. The use of nonpharmacologic techniques to prevent postoperative nausea and vomiting: a meta-analysis. *Anesth Analg* 1999;**88**:1362–9.
29. Eberhart LH, Morin AM, Bothner U, Georgieff M. Droperidol and 5-HT$_3$-receptor antagonists, alone or in combination, for prophylaxis of postoperative nausea and vomiting: a meta-analysis of randomised controlled trials. *Acta Anaesthesiol Scand* 2000;**44**:1252–7.
30. Tramèr MR, Reynolds DJM, Moore RA, McQuay HJ. When placebo controlled trials are essential and equivalence trials are inadequate. *BMJ* 1998;**317**:780–5.
31. Domino KB, Anderson EA, Polissar NL, Posner KL. Comparative efficacy and safety of ondansetron, droperidol, and metoclopramide for preventing postoperative nausea and vomiting: a meta-analysis. *Anesth Analg* 1999;**88**:1370–9.
32. Loewen PS, Marra CA, Zed PJ. 5-HT$_3$ receptor antagonists vs traditional agents for the prophylaxis of postoperative nausea and vomiting. *Can J Anaesth* 2000;**47**:1008–18.
33. Tramèr M, Moore A, McQuay H. Meta-analytic comparison of prophylactic antiemetic efficacy for postoperative nausea and vomiting: propofol anaesthesia *vs* omitting nitrous oxide *vs* a total i.v. anaesthesia with propofol. *Br J Anaesth* 1997;**78**:256–9.
34. Tramèr MR, Reynolds DJM, Moore RA, McQuay HJ. Impact of covert duplicate publication on meta-analysis: a case study. *BMJ* 1997;**315**:635–40.
35. Tramèr MR, Phillips C, Reynolds DJM, Moore RA, McQuay HJ. Cost-effectiveness of ondansetron for postoperative nausea and vomiting. *Anaesthesia* 1999;**54**:226–35.
36. Figueredo E, Canosa LG. Prevention or treatment of postoperative vomiting using ondansetron? A mathematical assessment. *J Clin Anesth* 1999;**11**:24–31.
37. Figueredo E, Canosa L. Prophylactic ondansetron for postoperative emesis: meta-analysis of its effectiveness in patients with previous history of postoperative nausea and vomiting. *Acta Anaesthesiol Scand* 1999;**43**:637–44.
38. Figueredo E, Canosa L. Prophylactic ondansetron for post-operative emesis: meta-analysis of its effectiveness in patients with and without a previous history of motion sickness. *Eur J Anaesthesiol* 1999;**16**:556–64.

39. Aspinall RL, Goodman NW. Denial of effective treatment and poor quality of clinical information in placebo controlled trials of ondansetron for postoperative nausea and vomiting: a review of published trials. *BMJ* 1995;**311**:844–6.
40. Kranke P, Apfel CC, Eberhart LH, Georgieff M, Roewer N. The influence of a dominating centre on a quantitative systematic review of granisetron for preventing postoperative nausea and vomiting. *Acta Anaesthesiol Scand* 2001;**45**: 659–70.
41. Kazemi-Kjellberg F, Henzi I, Tramèr MR. Treatment of established postoperative nausea and vomiting: a quantitative systematic review. *BMC Anesthesiol* 2001;**1**:2.
42. Tramèr MR. A rational approach to the control of postoperative nausea and vomiting: evidence from systematic reviews. Part II. Recommendations for prevention and treatment, and research agenda. *Acta Anaesthesiol Scand* 2001;**14**–9.
43. Gan TJ, Meyer T, Apfel CC, *et al.* Consensus guidelines for the management of postoperative nausea and vomiting. *Anesth Analg* (in press).
44. Palazzo M, Evans R. Logistic regression analysis of fixed patient factors for postoperative sickness: a model for risk assessment. *Br J Anaesth* 1993;**70**:135–40.
45. Haigh CG, Kaplan LA, Durham JM, Dupeyron JP, Harmer M, Kenny GN. Nausea and vomiting after gynaecological surgery: a meta-analysis of factors affecting their incidence. *Br J Anaesth* 1993;**71**:517–22.
46. Cohen MM, Duncan PG, De Boer DP, Tweed WA. The postoperative interview: assessing risk factors for nausea and vomiting. *Anesth Analg* 1994;**78**:7–16.
47. Apfel CC, Greim CA, Haubitz I, *et al.* A risk score to predict the probability of postoperative vomiting in adults. *Acta Anaesthesiol Scand* 1998;**42**:495–501.
48. Sinclair DR, Chung F, Mezei G. Can postoperative nausea and vomiting be predicted? *Anesthesiology* 1999;**91**:109–18.
49. Eberhart LH, Morin AM, Georgieff M. The menstruation cycle in the postoperative phase: its effect on the incidence of nausea and vomiting. *Anaesthesist* 2000;**49**:532–5.
50. Kranke P, Apfel CC, Papenfuss T, *et al.* An increased body mass index is no risk factor for postoperative nausea and vomiting: a systematic review and results of original data. *Acta Anaesthesiol Scand* 2001;**45**:160–6.
51. Eberhart LH, Hogel J, Seeling W, Staack AM, Geldner G, Georgieff M. Evaluation of three risk scores to predict postoperative nausea and vomiting. *Acta Anaesthesiol Scand* 2000;**44**:480–8.
52. Sweeney BP. Why does smoking protect against PONV? *Br J Anaesth* 2002;**89**:810–3.
53. Stadler M, Bardiau F, Seidel L, Albert A, Boogaerts JG. Difference in risk factors for postoperative nausea and vomiting. *Anesthesiology* 2003;**98**:46–52.
54. Møiniche S, Rømsing J, Dahl JB, Tramèr MR. Nonsteroidal antiinflammatory drugs and the risk of operative site bleeding after tonsillectomy: a quantitative systematic review. *Anesth Analg* 2003;**96**:68–77.
55. Tramèr MR, Carroll D, Campbell FA, Reynolds DJ, Moore RA, McQuay HJ. Cannabinoids for control of chemotherapy induced nausea and vomiting: quantitative systematic review. *BMJ* 2001;**323**:16–21.
56. Walder B, Schafer M, Henzi I, Tramèr MR. Efficacy and safety of patient-controlled opioid analgesia for acute postoperative pain: a quantitative systematic review. *Acta Anaesthesiol Scand* 2001;**45**:795–804.
57. Culebras X, Corpataux JD, Gaggero G, Tramèr MR. The antiemetic efficacy of droperidol added to morphine-PCA: a randomized, controlled, multicenter, dose-finding study. *Anesth Analg* (in press).

9: Propofol for anaesthesia and sedation

BERNHARD WALDER, MARTIN R TRAMÈR

Since its introduction in 1980, propofol (2,6-di-isopropylphenol)[1] has become a popular intravenous drug for anaesthesia, and for sedation in ophthalmology, interventional radiology, and endoscopical procedures, and in the intensive care unit. The number of patients that receive propofol can only be estimated. In France (population ~60 million), for instance, about 10 anaesthetic procedures per 100 inhabitants were performed in 1996.[2] If we assume that 40% of all anaesthesia and sedation is done using propofol, then propofol is given to about two million patients per year in France alone.

Propofol has several pharmacological advantages. It has a short duration of action related to a rapid redistribution (redistribution half-life, 13·4 min), a lack of prolonged sedation despite a long elimination half-life of 7·8 hours,[3] and a metabolic profile that appears to be independent of hepatic function.[4] No change in kinetic parameters has been reported in patients with renal and hepatic dysfunction. Thus, this hypnotic can be titrated easily, even in patients with renal or hepatic diseases. Propofol has multiple actions on the gamma-amino-butyric acid (GABA$_A$) receptor.[5] However, compared with midazolam, propofol seems to induce amnesia only rarely.[6]

In February 2003, a search in Medline using the keyword "propofol" yielded 6796 references. When the search was limited to review, 356 references remained. This large number of reviews suggests that propofol has gained widespread popularity among healthcare providers. A large majority of these articles, however, are on conventional narrative overviews. Systematic reviews provide more concise summaries on efficacy and harm of healthcare interventions (Chapter 3). Thus, this chapter will concentrate on systematic reviews on propofol's beneficial and harmful effects.

Methods

We searched for relevant reviews that reported on a reproducible systematic search strategy with predefined inclusion and exclusion criteria. A comprehensive search was conducted in Medline (last access 26 December 2002) using a recommended search algorithm for systematic reviews[7] and the keyword "propofol". We also screened our electronically accessible in-house database of systematically searched systematic reviews that are relevant to perioperative medicine (http://www.hcuge.ch/anesthesie/anglais/evidence/arevusyst.htm). The titles on this list are from regular searches in electronic databases (Medline, Cochrane Library), from contact with authors, and from hand searching of locally available anaesthesia journals. Finally, bibliographies of eligible reviews were scanned for further relevant papers.

Results

We identified 14 reports that could be regarded as systematic reviews according to our pre-hoc definition.[8-21] All were published in English, between 1995 and 2002; 10 were published in five anaesthesia journals, two in two neurological journals, one in a critical care journal, and one in a general medical journal.

Beneficial effects of propofol

Nine systematic reviews addressed mainly potentially beneficial effects of propofol: induction characteristics,[10] quality of recovery after anaesthesia,[9,14] prevention of postoperative nausea and vomiting,[15,17,18] and quality of sedation.[11,12,20]

Induction of anaesthesia

One systematic review compared propofol with sevoflurane for induction of anaesthesia.[10] Twelve randomised controlled trials with data on 1082 patients were analysed. The incidence of transient apnoea during induction was more frequent with propofol (33%) compared with sevoflurane (7%). The incidence of postoperative nausea and vomiting was halved when propofol was used for induction compared with sevoflurane. For all other tested end points – for instance, success rate of laryngeal mask insertion or patient satisfaction – there was no difference between the two methods of induction. The authors concluded that propofol may be preferable due to the lower incidence of postoperative nausea and vomiting, and because there was a trend towards an improved patient satisfaction.

Recovery from anaesthesia

Two systematic reviews investigated recovery from anaesthesia with propofol compared with inhalational agents. One review compared propofol with desflurane, and included six randomised controlled trials with data from 229 patients.[9] Another compared propofol with sevoflurane and included seven randomised controlled trials with data from 922 patients.[14] In both reviews, the average time to follow commands after extubation was slightly shorter with propofol than with the inhalational agents. The average time in the first review was 0·7 min, which was concluded not to be clinically relevant by the authors.[9] In the second review, the authors concluded that the time difference of 3·0 min was clinically relevant.[14]

Postoperative nausea and vomiting

Three systematic reviews studied the potentially beneficial effect of propofol on postoperative nausea and vomiting. One compared propofol with different anaesthesia regimens,[17] and analysed 84 randomised trials with data on 6069 patients. Propofol was shown to decrease the incidence of nausea and vomiting but only in patients with a high baseline risk of nausea and vomiting, only when propofol was used for both induction and maintenance of anaesthesia, and only in the immediate postoperative period. Compared with a non-propofol anaesthetic, the number needed to treat (NNT) to prevent nausea and vomiting within six hours after surgery was about five. The authors concluded that a propofol anaesthetic might be a useful choice in patients who were at high risk of postoperative nausea and vomiting. In a subsequent analysis, propofol was compared with omitting nitrous oxide[18] – another anaesthesia technique that has been shown to decrease the risk of postoperative nausea and vomiting (Chapter 8). Both strategies were shown to be equally effective in decreasing the incidence of postoperative vomiting; only propofol, however, had a positive impact on postoperative nausea. The third systematic review was sponsored by the manufacturer of propofol.[15] In this analysis, the NNT to prevent postoperative nausea and vomiting with propofol compared with inhalational agents was only about seven. Nevertheless, the authors concluded that this degree of efficacy was clinically relevant.

Sedation in critically ill patients

Three systematic reviews investigated sedation with propofol in mechanically ventilated patients. One review compared the sedation characteristics of propofol with several other hypnotics, including midazolam; it included 20 randomised controlled trials with data from 1863 patients.[12] The two remaining reviews compared propofol with midazolam; they included 17 randomised controlled trials (no information on the number of analysed patients was provided),[11] and 27 randomised controlled trials with data on 1624 patients,[20] respectively. The authors of all three reviews concluded that effective and adequate sedation in mechanically ventilated patients was possible with both propofol and midazolam, and that times to extubation were, on average, shorter with propofol. One review concluded that weaning times were shorter with propofol but only in patients who had received sedation for less than 36 hours.[20] There was an increased risk of arterial hypotension (number needed to harm (NNH), 12)[12,20] and of hypertriglyceridaemia (NNH, 6)[20] with propofol. None of the reviews was clearly in favour of one particular sedation technique in these patients.

Harmful effects of propofol

Five systematic reviews dealt mainly with adverse effects of propofol: pain on injection,[13] bradycardia,[16] and convulsion or seizure-like phenomena.[8,19,21]

Pain on injection

One systematic review compared the analgesic efficacy of interventions that were used to prevent a typical and well known, but poorly understood, adverse effect of propofol – that is, pain on injection.[13] Fifty-six randomised controlled trials with data on 6264 patients, testing 15 drugs (for instance, opioids or non-steroidal ant-inflammatory drugs (NSAIDs)), 12 physical measurements (for instance, warming or cooling of propofol), and combinations were analysed. On average, 70% of control patients who did not receive any analgesic intervention reported pain on injection. The most efficacious intervention was intravenous lidocaine 0·5 mg/kg, given as a Bier's block with a rubber tourniquet on the forearm for 30 seconds before injection of propofol; using this technique, the NNT to prevent pain compared with doing nothing was < 2. The authors concluded that this intervention should be used because it was simple, cheap, and efficacious, and that no further trials were needed in this setting.

Bradycardia

One systematic review investigated bradycardia and cardiac arrest in association with propofol anaesthesia.[16] Published and unpublished data on 32 182 patients from 17 randomised controlled trials, 31 case series, and 17 case reports were analysed. In the randomised trials, the additional risk of bradycardia with propofol compared with a non-propofol anaesthetic was approximately 9% (NNH, 11). In particular, children undergoing squint repair were shown to be at risk of bradycardia due to the oculocardiac reflex and despite prophylactic anticholinergics. It was estimated that one in 660 patients receiving a propofol anaesthetic may have a cardiac arrest who would not have had one had they not received propofol. The authors concluded that propofol should be used with caution in patients with conduction abnormalities, in those taking drugs to lower heart rate, in children undergoing strabismus surgery, in patients undergoing laparoscopies, in very sick and very old patients, and in young children.

Convulsion and seizure-like phenomena

Three systematic reviews addressed the question as to whether propofol had proconvulsive or anticonvulsive properties. One compared propofol with methohexital for electroconvulsive therapy in 15 randomised controlled trials with data on 706 patients.[19] The duration of motor seizure was shorter with propofol (weighted mean difference, 8·4 seconds). The clinical relevance of this difference remained unclear; data on clinical outcome were sparse and inconclusive. These trials do not provide evidence that propofol had anticonvulsive properties as methohexital, the comparator drug, is proconvulsive. The second systematic review was on the treatment of refractory status epilepticus with propofol, pentobarbital, or midazolam.[8] Twenty-eight observational studies and case series (there were no randomised trials) with data on 193 patients were analysed. Suppression of the EEG was shown to be possible with all three drugs. The authors suggested that not the drug *per se* but suppression of EEG background was important for the treatment of refractory status epilepticus. The third systematic review analysed reports on seizure-like phenomena in patients who had received propofol.[21] Eighty-one observational reports (no randomised trials could be retrieved) with data on 81 patients with or without pre-existing epilepsy were analysed. Seizure-like phenomena occurred most often at induction or at emergence of anaesthesia or sedation with propofol. The authors suggested that a change in the cerebral concentration of propofol might be causal for these phenomena occurring together.

Discussion

Propofol is a widely used intravenous hypnotic. It has gained popularity due to its favourable pharmacokinetics and since early studies suggested that the incidence of postoperative nausea and vomiting was decreased compared with conventional volatile-based anaesthesia. However, reports on potentially lethal haemodynamic instability, progressive myocardial failure, cardiac dysrhythmia, rhabdomyolysis, metabolic acidosis, and hyperkalaemia in relation to propofol have dampened the initial euphoria.[22] Impaired fatty acid oxidation with failure of the mitochondrial respiratory chain at complex 11, mimicking mitochondrial myopathies, has been proposed as an origin of this syndrome.[23] There is also an increased risk of bloodstream infection with the use of propofol.[24,25] Thus, as for all drugs, it is important for rational decision making that all valid data on the benefit and harm of propofol are gathered systematically, and that rational conclusions are reached that are based on the highest possible level of evidence.

We unearthed a large number of narrative conventional review articles on propofol. Eventually, we found 14 reports that were on systematic reviews, and were therefore valid for the purpose of this overview. This is still an amazingly large number and it perhaps reflects the interest that propofol has gained among physicians and researchers. Although some of the reviews (for instance, those on postoperative nausea and vomiting) overlapped, we may assume that data from more than 50 000 patients have been critically appraised and qualitatively and quantitatively analysed in these reports. Nine systematic reviews dealt primarily with potentially beneficial effects of propofol. There is strong evidence that awakening times after both sedation and anaesthesia are shorter with propofol compared with other hypnotics or with some inhalational anaesthetics. The clinical relevance of these differences, however, remains obscure. After anaesthesia, the differences in awakening times are in the order of minutes, and this is unlikely to be of any clinical relevance. In patients who are mechanically ventilated and sedated for several days, average weaning times with propofol are no different from those with midazolam, and with both drugs there is a wide variability in weaning times. When sedation lasts for less than 36 hours, weaning times with propofol are, on average, 2·2 hours shorter than with midazolam; some may regard this as a clinically relevant benefit of propofol.

The incidence of postoperative nausea and vomiting is lower when propofol is used. Thus, together with other choices, a propofol anaesthetic may be regarded as part of a rational strategy to decrease the baseline risk of postoperative nausea and vomiting (Chapter 8). However, propofol should not be seen as a universal anti-emetic drug; at least five high-risk patients need to receive a propofol anaesthetic for one not to vomit or not to be nauseous who would have done so had they all received a non-propofol anaesthetic. Also, this beneficial effect is short lived – it is unlikely to last longer than six hours after surgery. More enthusiastic conclusions, despite higher NNTs (that is, despite less benefit),[15] are likely to be biased in favour of propofol as these analyses were sponsored by the manufacturer of propofol.

These systematic reviews did not ignore risk. Five reports were primarily on risk and some of the others included information on harm. Compared with volatile anaesthetics, propofol increases the likelihood of apnoea during induction,[10] and of bradycardia during anesthesia.[16] When used for long-term sedation, there is an increased risk of hypertriglyceridaemia and of arterial hypotension.[20] Finally, an annoying and well known adverse effect of this drug is pain on injection.[13] Physicians who are using propofol need to be aware of these potential adverse effects. Pain on injection, for instance, is a minor, almost trivial, adverse effect and the most effective analgesic intervention to prevent it, a lidocaine Bier's block, is simple to use. None of these adverse effects really limits the use of propofol as long as physicians know how to prevent them and how to deal with them once they have occurred. As with other drugs, a contraindication to using propofol is the absence of an indication.

Perhaps the issue associated with the most uncertainty here was the use of propofol and its relation to convulsions. There is still no consensus as to whether propofol should be used in patients with epilepsy (for instance, those undergoing surgery for epilepsy). Uncontrolled observations suggest that convulsions or seizure-like phenomena may occur in patients with or without epilepsy who are receiving propofol. Propofol has been used for the treatment of refractory status epilepticus. However, no single randomised trial exists in this setting. Another related setting where propofol is presumably often used, despite a lack of valid data that support its usefulness, is in acute brain injury with subsequent increased intracranial pressure. This pathology has become epidemic in young men.[26] As for the treatment of refractory status epilepticus, the role of propofol in these patients is unclear. The lack of valid data on the role of propofol in epileptic or brain-injured patients raises ethical concerns. The use of the anaesthetic propofol as an antiepileptic drug is off-label and should be supported by valid scientific data. Interestingly, the manufacturer of propofol did not seem to show much interest in these questions.

A major limitation of all these systematic reviews (or more precisely, of the original studies) was that mostly surrogate end points were analysed. For instance, there were numerous investigations on time of recovery after anaesthesia or sedation; however, only rarely was the depth of anaesthesia or sedation reported. Also, trials on postoperative nausea and vomiting almost never reported on the postoperative nutrition of patients, length of hospital stay, unanticipated hospitalisation due to intractable vomiting, or supplemental workload of nurses due to the vomiting (time for cleaning, for instance).

In conclusion, a propofol anaesthetic reduces the incidence of postoperative nausea and vomiting in the short term compared with volatile anaesthetics. Anaesthetists may make use of this characteristic as part of a multimodal strategy to control postoperative nausea and vomiting. Differences in induction and recovery characteristics compared with volatile anaesthetics are, however, of doubtful clinical relevance. Propofol has probably both proconvulsive and anticonvulsive properties, and its use in patients with epilepsy remains controversial. Well known adverse effects of propofol are pain on injection, arterial hypotension and bradycardia, and, when used for long-term sedation in critically ill patients, hypertriglyceridaemia.

123

References

1. Rogers KM, Dewar KM, McCubbin TD, Spence AA. Preliminary experience with ICI 35 868 as an i.v. induction agent: comparison with althesin. *Br J Anaesth* 1980;**52**:807–10.
2. Clergue F, Auroy Y, Pequignot F, Jougla E, Lienhart A, Laxenaire MC. French survey of anesthesia in 1996. *Anesthesiology* 1999;**91**:1509–20.
3. McMurray TJ, Collier PS, Carson IW, Lyons SM, Elliott P. Propofol sedation after open heart surgery: a clinical and pharmacokinetic study. *Anaesthesia* 1990;**45**:322–6.
4. Lange H, Stephan H, Rieke H, Kellermann M, Sonntag H, Bircher J. Hepatic and extrahepatic disposition of propofol in patients undergoing coronary bypass surgery. *Br J Anaesth* 1990;**64**:563–70.
5. Bai D, Pennefather PS, MacDonald JF, Orser BA. The general anesthetic propofol slows deactivation and desensitization of GABA(A) receptors. *J Neurosci* 1999;**19**:10635–46.
6. Weinbroum AA, Halpern P, Rudick V, Sorkine P, Freedman M, Geller E. Midazolam versus propofol for long-term sedation in the ICU: a randomized prospective comparison. *Intensive Care Med* 1997;**23**:1258–63.
7. Hunt DL, McKibbon KA. Locating and appraising systematic review. *Ann Intern Med* 1997;**126**:532–8.
8. Claassen J, Hirsch LJ, Emerson RG, Mayer SA. Treatment of refractory status epilepticus with pentobarbital, propofol, or midazolam: a systematic review. *Epilepsia* 2002;**43**:146–53.
9. Dexter F, Tinker JH. Comparisons between desflurane and isoflurane or propofol on time to following commands and time to discharge: a metaanalysis. *Anesthesiology* 1995;**83**:77–82.
10. Joo HS, Perks WJ. Sevoflurane versus propofol for anesthetic induction: a meta-analysis. *Anesth Analg* 2000;**91**:213–9.
11. Magarey JM. Propofol or midazolam – which is best for the sedation of adult ventilated patients in intensive care units? A systematic review. *Aust Crit Care* 2001;**14**:147–54.
12. Ostermann ME, Keenan SP, Seiferling RA, Sibbald WJ. Sedation in the intensive care unit: a systematic review. *JAMA* 2000;**283**:1451–9.
13. Picard P, Tramèr MR. Prevention of pain on injection with propofol: a quantitative systematic review. *Anesth Analg* 2000;**90**:963–9.
14. Robinson BJ, Uhrich TD, Ebert TJ. A review of recovery from sevoflurane anaesthesia: comparisons with isoflurane and propofol including meta-analysis. *Acta Anaesthesiol Scand* 1999;**43**:185–90.
15. Sneyd JR, Carr A, Byrom WD, Bilski AJ. A meta-analysis of nausea and vomiting following maintenance of anaesthesia with propofol or inhalational agents. *Eur J Anaesthesiol* 1998;**15**:433–5.
16. Tramèr MR, Moore RA, McQuay HJ. Propofol and bradycardia: causation, frequency and severity. *Br J Anaesth* 1997;**78**:642–51.
17. Tramèr M, Moore A, McQuay H. Meta-analytic comparison of prophylactic antiemetic efficacy for postoperative nausea and vomiting: propofol anaesthesia vs omitting nitrous oxide vs total i.v. anaesthesia with propofol. *Br J Anaesth* 1997;**78**:256–9.
18. Tramèr M, Moore A, McQuay H. Propofol anaesthesia and postoperative nausea and vomiting: quantitative systematic review of randomized controlled studies. *Br J Anaesth* 1997;**78**:247–55.
19. Walder B, Seeck M, Tramèr MR. Propofol versus methohexital for electroconvulsive therapy: a meta-analysis. *J Neurosurg Anesthesiol* 2001;**13**:93–8.
20. Walder B, Elia N, Henzi I, Romand JR, Tramèr MR. A lack of evidence of superiority of propofol versus midazolam for sedation in mechanically ventilated critically ill patients: a qualitative and quantitative systematic review. *Anesth Analg* 2001;**92**:975–83.
21. Walder B, Tramèr MR, Seeck M. Seizure-like phenomena and propofol: a systematic review. *Neurology* 2002;**58**:1327–32.

22. Cremer OL, Moons KG, Bouman EA, Kruijswijk JE, de Smet AM, Kalkman CJ. Long-term propofol infusion and cardiac failure in adult head-injured patients. *Lancet* 2001;**357**:117–8.
23. Wolf A, Weir P, Segar P, Stone J, Shield J. Impaired fatty acid oxidation in propofol infusion syndrome. *Lancet* 2001;**357**:606–7.
24. Bennett SN, McNeil MM, Bland LA, *et al*. Postoperative infections traced to contamination of an intravenous anesthetic, propofol. *N Engl J Med* 1995;**333**: 147–54.
25. Kuehnert MJ, Webb RM, Jochimsen EM, *et al*. Staphylococcus aureus bloodstream infections among patients undergoing electroconvulsive therapy traced to breaks in infection control and possible extrinsic contamination by propofol. *Anesth Analg* 1997;**85**:420–5.
26. Murray CJ, Lopez AD. Mortality by cause for eight regions of the world: Global Burden of Disease Study. *Lancet* 1997;**349**:1269–76.

10: Preventing central venous catheter related complications

MEHRENGISE K COOPER,
ADRIENNE G RANDOLPH

Central venous catheters (CVCs) are often required for optimal perioperative care. They are used for the infusion of specific drugs (for example, vasopressors), blood products, maintenance fluids, parenteral nutrition, haemodynamic monitoring, and/or blood sampling. CVCs are placed percutaneously into central veins (subclavian, internal jugular, or femoral); the size and length used depend on the size of the patient. The placement and maintenance of CVCs are frequently associated with iatrogenic complications. Pneumothorax, haemothorax, nerve injury, line malplacement, and arrhythmias can occur during placement. The most common maintenance complication is CVC related bloodstream infection, with reported rates of up to 12·1%.[1] Other infective complications are endocarditis, septic thrombophlebitis, and metastatic infections. Thrombotic complications are also common. Deep venous thrombosis occurs in up to 21·5% of cases and can lead to pulmonary embolism, thrombophlebitis, and an inability to cannulate the vein when future access is required.

CVC infection is one of the leading causes of nosocomial bloodstream infections. Nosocomial infections are associated with an increased length of hospital and intensive care unit (ICU) stay, hospital costs and attributable mortality. Pittet *et al.*[2] reported an attributable mortality rate of 35% (95% confidence interval 25% to 45%) in a group of critically ill patients on a surgical ICU from nosocomial blood stream infection related to CVC infections and pneumonia. Reporting for the ICU–Bacteremia Study Group, Renaud and Brun-Buisson showed that in 28 patients with definite CVC related bacteraemia, the attributable mortality was 11·5%.[3] DiGiovine and colleagues found no excess mortality in ICU patients following bloodstream infection compared with matched controls, but they did report that overall, bloodstream infections led to an extra five-day stay on the ICU with an excess cost of $16 000.[4] A recent systematic audit reviewing economic evidence and nosocomial infection reported that costs attributable to bloodstream infection across studies averaged $38 703.[5] In summary, it is clear that CVC related infections are associated with high patient morbidity and considerable additional expense.

The majority of iatrogenic complications associated with CVCs can be prevented. A large body of solid evidence exists showing that CVC infections can be markedly reduced to minimal levels with meticulous care. Placement complications can also be reduced with technological support for visualisation. Using data from randomised controlled trials and systematic reviews, a set of guidelines has been published in the United States by the Centers for Disease Control and Prevention (CDC) and Healthcare Infection Control Practices Advisory Committee (HICPAC) for the prevention of CVC related infections. This chapter will summarise the most recent HICPAC compilation of evidence and discuss the following important issues: full asepsis for CVC placement and management, types of CVC (antiseptic-impregnated and antibiotic-impregnated), site of CVC placement, ultrasound to guide CVC placement, tunnelling of CVCs, heparin and heparin-bonded CVCs, occlusive dressings, and CVC-replacement strategies. Other CVC management topics are discussed in depth in the HICPAC review.[6]

Identifying central venous catheter related infection

CVC related bloodstream infection has been defined as bacteraemia/fungaemia in a patient with a CVC with at least one positive blood culture obtained from a peripheral vein, clinical manifestations of infections (fever, chills, and/or hypotension), and no apparent source for the bloodstream infection except the CVC. One of the following should be present:

- a positive semiquantitative (>15 colony forming units (CFU)/catheter segment), or quantitative (>10^3 CFU/catheter segment culture) culture, whereby the same organism is isolated from the catheter segment and peripheral blood
- simultaneous quantitative blood cultures with a >5:1 ratio central venous access versus peripheral, or
- a differential period of central venous catheter culture versus blood culture positivity of >2 hours.

The most commonly used definition requires culturing the CVC tip, and this requires removing the CVC. A common clinical practice is to draw a culture through the CVC, possibly start antibiotics through the CVC if the clinical status of the patient warrants it, and remove the CVC if the culture is positive and send the CVC tip for culture at that time. Without a quantitative comparison of CVC and peripheral cultures, it may not be clear that the CVC is the actual infection source. Therefore, it is important to draw simultaneous peripheral blood cultures whenever possible. Because the majority of fevers in hospitalised patients are not associated with bloodstream infections, removal of CVCs with every temperature spike will result in a large number of unnecessary CVC replacements.

Unfortunately, management strategies for suspected CVC infection have not been as thoroughly studied as have strategies to prevent CVC related complications. The actual diagnosis of CVC related bloodstream infections can be difficult, leading some institutions to report CVC associated bloodstream infection rates defined as the number of patients who have bacteraemia with a CVC in place. Although this rate will overestimate the actual number of CVC related bloodstream infections, a definition of CVC related infections based on CVC tip cultures may underestimate the actual number of infections. For benchmarking purposes, an institution should report the number of CVC associated bloodstream infections per 1000 CVC days (CVC days are the total number of days of exposure to CVCs by all patients in the selected population during the selected time period) and also assess the number of central venous CVC related infections by careful scrutiny of the charts of all patients with bloodstream infections and assessment of CVC tip cultures when performed.

Full asepsis for central venous catheter placement and management

Full asepsis includes good hand hygiene and proper aseptic technique with maximal sterile barrier precautions.[7] Before gloving, hands must be washed with an antibacterial soap and water or with a waterless alcohol based product. A full patient drape should be used to minimise any chance of contamination during placement.

Cleaning the skin before inserting a CVC is essential, and povidone–iodine is one of the most widely used antiseptics for this purpose. Chlorhexidine is a germicide widely used for disinfection. One randomised controlled trial comparing 2% chlorhexidine with 10% povidone–iodine for cutaneous disinfection before placement of central venous and arterial access showed a reduction of infection in the group using chlorhexidine.[8] Another group comparing 10% povidone–iodine with 0·5% chlorhexidine showed no difference between the two agents for the prevention of CVC related bloodstream infection.[9] Skin cleansing is of paramount importance using one of the standard agents available.

By using strict guidelines to manage CVCs in critically ill patients, Eggiman and colleagues reduced the episodes of bloodstream infection from 22·9 to 6·2 episodes per 1000 CVC days.[10] The interventions used included strict sterile technique, specific CVC care, and operator training. This suggests that, by using correct hand hygiene and using meticulous care, infection rates can be reduced.

The clinical bottom line: Hand washing and maximal sterile barrier precautions, together with skin cleansing using either 2% chlorhexidine, tincture of iodine, or 70% alcohol are essential to reduce the risk of CVC related bloodstream infection when obtaining central venous access. Devotion to meticulous CVC care results in reduced infection rates.

Antiseptic-impregnated central venous catheters

In searching for methods to reduce the incidence of nosocomial infections associated with the placement of central venous lines, CVCs impregnated with an external surface antiseptic coating of chlorhexidine–silver sulfadiazine were designed to reduce the incidence of CVC related bloodstream infection by inhibiting bacterial colonisation of the CVC surface.[11] In a meta-analysis reported by Veenstra and colleagues, 2830 CVCs were studied in a total of 13 randomised/quasi-randomised controlled trials where chlorhexidine–silver sulfadiazine impregnated on the external surface of CVCs were evaluated in the prevention of CVC related bloodstream infection.[12] Twelve studies were used in the analysis of CVC colonisation and 11 in the analysis of CVC related bloodstream infection. One-third of the patients were admitted to the ICU; the remainder were from other hospital settings. There was no significant difference in CVC location between the two groups assessed, where the site of CVC was reported. There was a reduction in the risk for CVC colonisation and CVC related bloodstream infection in the antiseptic impregnated group.

In a separate report, Veenstra and colleagues reviewed the clinical and economic outcomes and, by using a decision analytic model, compared the short-term use (2–10 days) of chlorhexidine–silver sulfadiazine-impregnated multi-lumen CVCs with nonimpregnated CVCs.[13] Data from randomised controlled trials, meta-analyses, and case–control studies were included. It was found that the use of antiseptic-impregnated CVCs in patients at high risk for CVC related bloodstream infection was associated with reduced medical care costs, a reduction in the incidence of CVC related bloodstream infection, and a decrease in the incidence of death. Analysis suggested that for every 300 lines used, $59 000 would be saved, seven cases of CVC related bloodstream infection would be avoided, and one death prevented.

The longer-term benefit of the placement of these CVCs requires more study. The half-life of the antiseptic used has been shown to decrease with time. Walder and colleagues recently performed a meta-analysis reviewing trials where anti-infective coating or cuffing was used to reduce the risk of infection.[14] In five trials where chlorhexidine–silver sulfadiazine coating was used (1269 CVCs), the average insertion time was a median of six days (range 5·2–7·5 days) and the risk of bloodstream infection was reduced from 4·1% to 1·9% in the group where anti-infective CVCs were placed. In a further five trials (1544 CVCs), where the average insertion time was a median of 12 days (range 7·8–20 days), the risk of bloodstream infection was 4·5% in the control group, compared with 4·2% in the group where the anti-infective CVCs had been used.

In addition, the US Food and Drug Administration has raised concern over the rare cases of hypersensitivity reported following the use of these CVCs and other devices impregnated with chlorhexidine–silver sulfadiazine. In children there are no recommendations regarding the use of these CVCs and more work is needed to evaluate this population.

The clinical bottom line: CVCs with antiseptic coating are of benefit and are cost effective for short-term use in patients at high risk for sepsis.

Antibiotic-impregnated central venous catheters

In addition to antiseptic coatings on CVCs, lines impregnated with antibiotics have also been developed to combat CVC related bloodstream infection following nosocomial colonisation. In a randomised controlled trial, Raad et al. assessed the efficacy of CVCs coated with minocycline and rifampicin (both internal and external coating).[15] These broad-spectrum antibiotics are not routinely used to treat bloodstream infection and were chosen to minimise the likelihood of developing antibiotic resistance. A total of 281 patients in five centres were studied. CVC related bloodstream infections developed in 5% and 0% of patients in which uncoated CVCs (controls) and coated CVCs, respectively, were used; colonisation occurred in 26% of the uncoated group and 8% of the coated group. The median time for duration of CVC placement was six days. The cost saving per surviving patient where a coated CVC was used was $724·35, and the use of these CVCs may assist in saving hospital costs.

There is no systematic review assessing antibiotic-impregnated CVCs. One randomised controlled trial has compared the rates of CVC colonisation and CVC related bloodstream infection in CVCs impregnated with minocycline and rifampicin and in CVCs impregnated with chlorhexidine–silver sulfadiazine.[16] All patients required central venous access for more than three days.

Minocycline–rifampicin CVCs were significantly more likely to prevent catheter related infections than antiseptic-coated CVCs.

Currently, the smallest-sized CVC available with antibiotic impregnation is 5F. These CVCs cannot be recommended for use in children as no trials have investigated their use in this age group. More work is therefore needed in this area.

The clinical bottom line: The use of antibiotic-impregnated CVCs reduced infection and is cost-effective in patients at high risk for sepsis. Antibiotic-impregnated CVCs are possibly superior to antiseptic-coated CVCs in preventing CVC related infection, but this may be dependent upon the patient population and the baseline rate of CVC infection.

Site of central venous catheter placement

The most frequently used anatomical sites for CVC insertion are the internal jugular and subclavian veins. Ruesch *et al.* reviewed the data from 17 prospective comparative non-randomised trials comparing internal jugular and subclavian CVCs.[17] In total, 2085 internal jugular vein and 2428 subclavian vein CVCs were used. In six trials (2010 catheters), the placement of subclavian CVCs was associated with a significantly increased incidence of arterial puncture; on the basis of this systematic searched data, of 39 attempts to access the internal jugular vein, one attempt will be associated with arterial puncture. Malpositioning of the device is associated more frequently with cannulation of the subclavian vein.

Using the femoral vein as the site for CVC placement is associated with a higher risk of infection compared with using the subclavian vein. In a randomised controlled trial by Merrer *et al.*, 289 patients underwent CVC placement into subclavian or femoral sites.[18] Placement of a CVC into the femoral vein was associated with a higher rate of infection (19·8% femoral, 4·5% subclavian) and thrombotic complications (21·5% femoral, 1·9% subclavian). In critically ill patients, the addition of an infection or thrombotic event is associated with significant morbidity. Thus, the subclavian vein is recommended over the femoral vein for CVC placement in adults.

The femoral vein is more commonly used in children as a site for the placement of a CVC. For children, the anatomical landmarks are easy to identify compared with approaches for internal jugular and subclavian veins. Of course, in children there is concern about the nappy area and the risk of soiling around the CVC insertion site. However, a prospective non-randomised study reviewing the complications of femoral and non-femoral CVCs revealed no significant difference in complication rates.[19] Because the rate of complications with femoral CVCs in children is reported to be low, use of the femoral vein for short-term access in children appears to be acceptable, but further study is needed to assess the risk of thrombosis and infection with the use of CVCs over seven days.

The clinical bottom line: The subclavian vein has the lowest incidence of reported infections in adults and is the vein of choice. In children, the femoral vein is acceptable for short-term central venous access.

Ultrasound to guide central venous catheter placement

The standard technique has used anatomical landmarks to guide the operator to correct CVC placement. These landmarks may not always correlate with correct vessel location. Two systematic reviews have looked at ultrasound in assisting the placement of CVCs. In a meta-analysis, Randolph et al. evaluated the effect of real-time ultrasound guidance using different ultrasound techniques used in CVC placement.[20] They looked at eight randomised controlled trials and found that ultrasound-guided CVC placement was of benefit. Ultrasound guidance significantly increases the probability of successful placement of CVC and reduces the number of complications encountered during CVC placement. It also reduces the need for multiple CVC placement. For example, by using ultrasound guidance in seven patients, one patient complication will be prevented; and using this technique in five patients will prevent more than one attempt at CVC insertion having to be made.

Keenan undertook a review of 18 controlled studies, all comparing the use of real-time ultrasound with using anatomical landmarks.[21] A significant reduction in placement failure rate, number of attempts at placement, and arterial punctures was seen where real-time ultrasound was used. In addition, in a subgroup analysis, by using external internal jugular probes for the internal jugular vein, outcomes were improved when used by a less experienced operator.

The clinical bottom line: Ultrasound is an extremely valuable tool for the placement of CVCs and minimises many placement complications, especially those with difficult access. It is a technique in which all operators should have experience.

Tunnelling of central venous catheters

As previously discussed, infections related to the use of short-term CVCs, especially in the critically ill, are the most common causes of

CVC related complication. The majority of these episodes are associated with CVC tip colonisation, with the site of cutaneous insertion being the entry port for microorganisms. By increasing the distance between a potentially unclean site and the entry site into the vein, tunnelling the CVC can potentially reduce the risk of CVC related infection.

Randolph *et al.* performed a meta-analysis critically reviewing seven randomised controlled trials where tunnelled CVCs were compared with standard placement.[22] The patient populations reviewed included adults and children who required CVCs in place for an average of up to 30 days. Tunnelling decreased bacterial colonisation of the catheter by 39% and decreased CVC related sepsis with bacteriological confirmation by 44% when compared with standard placement. The decrease in CVC related sepsis with bacteriological confirmation was largely due to a significant reduction in risk from a single trial with tunnelling at the site of the internal jugular vein. However, the risk reduction was not significant when pooling the results from the five trials using subclavian CVCs. This is an area where more work will be needed to further elucidate the use of tunnelled subclavian CVCs for long-term use.

The clinical bottom line: Tunnelling CVCs may reduce the risk of sepsis but more studies are needed before it can be recommended as a placement strategy for short-term central venous access.

Heparin and heparin bonded CVCs

Vascular thrombosis and subsequent systemic infection are well known to be associated with CVCs.[23] Although heparin is an effective anticoagulant, it is associated with risks including autoimmune-mediated heparin-induced thrombocytopenia, allergic reactions, and the potential for bleeding; it should not be used without clear evidence of benefit. A meta-analysis evaluating the effect of heparin on thrombus formation and infection in patients with CVCs and pulmonary artery catheters has been performed by Randolph *et al.*[24] The 14 randomised controlled trials evaluated both the use of heparin and the use of heparin bonded CVCs. Heparin bonding reduces the risk of clot formation within the first 24 hours following placement of pulmonary artery catheter and is standard on most commercially available pulmonary artery catheters. For other CVCs, the combined data showed that prophylactic heparin reduced the rate of CVC related vascular thrombosis and bacterial colonisation and may decrease CVC related bacteraemia. Unfortunately, the actual effective antithrombotic dose of heparin could not be extrapolated from the studies available.

In the meta-analysis reported above there was no information on heparin bonded CVCs in children. One randomised controlled trial evaluated the use of heparin bonded CVCs in the paediatric population.[25] A total of 209 patients (aged 0–16 years) were enrolled. Compared with non-heparin bonded CVCs, the use of heparin bonded CVCs resulted in a significant reduction in infection (positive blood culture heparin bonded 1%, non-heparin bonded 18%) and thrombosis (0% heparin bonded, 8% non-heparin bonded). The number of heparin bonded CVCs that would need to be used to avoid one episode of infection was three, and to avoid one episode of thrombosis the number was 13.

The clinical bottom line: Prophylactic heparin probably decreases the rate of CVC related thrombosis but the most effective dose of heparin is unclear. Heparin bonding has been shown to benefit pediatric patients but a confirmatory study is needed before recommending it as common practice.

Occlusive dressings

Securing the CVC in place is essential. Different dressings are available to assist with this. Transparent semipermeable polyurethane dressings allow the CVC site to be continually inspected, while providing an occlusive dressing. In a meta-analysis by Hoffmann and colleagues, seven studies comparing gauze and tape with transparent dressings were critically appraised.[26] There was an increased relative risk overall for CVC tip infection, but no increased risk for CVC related sepsis or bacteraemia using the transparent dressing. The recommendations advise that either sterile gauze or transparent, semipermeable dressing cover the CVC site. If the patient is diaphoretic, or if the site is oozing or bleeding, then a gauze dressing is preferable.

The clinical bottom line: Both gauze–tape and transparent dressings are acceptable. Use of ointments under the dressing is not recommended. Gauze and tape should be changed every two days and transparent dressings every seven days – sooner if they are soiled.

Central venous catheter exchange strategies

Replacement of CVCs can be achieved either by replacing the line in a new site or by exchanging the CVC over a guidewire. Cook and colleagues reviewed 12 randomised trials that compared the effect of guidewire exchange with new-site replacement on the incidence of CVC related infections and placement complications.[27] The guidewire exchange replacement strategy was associated with nonsignificant trends towards a higher rate of CVC infections. There were, overall, fewer complications associated with using a guidewire. Replacing

> **Box 10.1 The CDC/HICPAC system for categorising recommendations**
>
> - Category IA: Strongly recommended for implementation, supported by well designed studies (experimental, clinical, epidemiological)
> - Category IB: Strongly recommended for implementation, supported by some experimental, clinical or epidemiological studies, strong theoretic rationale
> - Category IC: Required by state or federal regulations, rules or standards
> - Category II: Suggestions for implementation, supported by suggestive clinical or epidemiological studies or theoretic rationale
> - Unresolved issue: Represents an unresolved issue for which the evidence is insufficient or no consensus regarding efficacy exists
>
> CDC = Centers for Disease Control and Prevention; HICPAC = Healthcare Infection Control Practices Advisory Committee

CVCs by either method every three days was of no benefit in preventing infections compared with replacing CVCs every seven days or on an as-needed basis.

The clinical bottom line: Use of a guidewire to exchange a malfunctioning CVC is acceptable but is not recommended as a routine strategy to prevent CVC related infection. Prophylactic replacement of CVC at new sites or via guidewire exchange every three days is not recommended.

Conclusions

In summary, CVCs are necessary for the management of many patients during the perioperative period. The use of these lines is not without significant risk for complications and morbidity, mainly from nosocomial CVC related bloodstream infection. Infectious complications can be minimised by using strict aseptic techniques for line placement with maximal sterile barrier precautions, by appropriate choice of site for placement, and by ensuring that these lines are cared for with strict aseptic technique. If these interventions do not result in an acceptably low CVC related infection rate, CVCs impregnated with antibiotics or with an antiseptic coating can be used.

Box 10.1 shows the CDC/HICPAC evidence-grading system for categorising these recommendations.[6] The HICPAC recommendations for the management of CVCs[6] are based on solid evidence and can be stated with a high degree of certainty. Future moves to minimise the morbidity and cost of associated complications will require strict adherence to these recommendations by physicians. Altering clinician practice is, unfortunately, exceptionally challenging.[28,29] Although meticulous attention to CVC management can be mundane, it has enormous pay-offs for the patient. Minimisation of CVC related infections is one indicator that should be more rigorously applied when evaluating the quality of care across institutions.

HICPAC recommendations for the management of central venous catheters

For patients who require central venous access as part of management in the operating room and in the ICU settings, these recommendations are listed below. All those listed are Category IA, IB, or II.

Hand hygiene

- Ensure proper hand hygiene by washing hands with antiseptic soap and water, or waterless alcohol-based preparations (IA).
- Palpation of the insertion site should not be performed after application of antiseptic, unless aseptic technique is maintained (IA).
- Use of gloves does not obviate the need for hand hygiene (IA).

Aseptic technique during CVC and care

- This is essential for insertion and care of the CVCs (IA).
- Wear sterile gloves for CVC insertion (IA).
- Maximal sterile barrier precautions should be used – cap, mask, sterile gown, sterile gloves, sterile full-body drapes (IA).

Cutaneous asepsis

- Ensure proper disinfection with appropriate antiseptic before CVC insertion, and during dressing changes (IA).
- Allow antiseptic to remain on the insertion site and allow air to dry before inserting CVC. Allow povidone–iodine to remain on the skin for at least two minutes if the surface is not dry (IB).

Central venous catheter selection

- Use a CVC with the minimum number of lumens needed for patient management (IB).
- Use an antibiotic or antiseptic-impregnated CVC in adults where the duration of use is expected to be more than five days if, after implementing a comprehensive strategy to reduce rates of CVC related bloodstream infection, the rate of infection is greater than the goals advised by the individual institution (IB).
- Personnel competent at placement should supervise trainees (IA).

Central venous catheter insertion site

- When choosing the placement site, balance risks against benefits for minimising both infectious complications and mechanical complications (IA).
- Use subclavian site in adults to reduce infection risk for nontunnelled CVC placement (IA).
- For the use of lines for hemodialysis and pharesis, place CVCs in femoral or jugular veins to avoid venous stenosis (IA).
- The femoral site is acceptable for short-term CVC placement in children (IA).

Catheter-site dressing regimens

- Use sterile gauze, or sterile transparent, semipermeable dressing to cover the CVC site (IA).
- Change dressings every week, depending upon individual patient circumstances (II).
- Replace dressing if it becomes damp, loosened, soiled or when insertion site is being inspected (IB).
- If the patient is diaphoretic, or if the site is oozing or bleeding, a gauze dressing is the preferred dressing (II).
- Do not use topical antibiotic ointment or cream on insertion sites, because of the risk of the promotion of fungal infection and antimicrobial resistance (IA).

Prophylactic antibiotics

- Do not administer antibiotic prophylaxis routinely to prevent CVC colonisation (IA).

References

1. Centers for Disease Control and Prevention. National Nosocomial Infections Surveillance (NNIS) System Report, Data Summary from January 1992–June 2001, Issued August 2001. *Am J Infect Control* 2001;**29**:404–21.
2. Pittet D, Tarara D, Wenzel RP. Nosocomial bloodstream infection in critically ill patients: excess length of stay, extra costs, and attributable mortality. *JAMA* 1994;**271**:1598–1601.
3. Renaud B, Brun-Buisson C, for the ICU–Bacteremia Study Group. Outcomes of primary and catheter-related bacteremia: a cohort and case–control study in critically ill patients. *Am J Resp Crit Care Med* 2001;**163**:1584–90.
4. DiGiovine B, Chenoweth C, Watts C, Higgins M. The attributable mortality and costs of primary nosocomial bloodstream infections in the intensive care unit. *Am J Respir Crit Care Med* 1999;**160**:976–81.
5. Stone PW, Larson E, Kawar LN. A systematic audit of economic evidence linking nosocomial infections and infection control interventions: 1990–2000. *Am J Infect Control* 2002;**30**:145–52.

6. O'Grady NP, Alexander M, Dellinger EP, *et al.* Guidelines for the prevention of intravascular catheter-related infections. *Pediatrics* 2002;**110(5)**:e51.
7. Raad II, Hohn DC, Gilbreath BJ, *et al.* Prevention of central venous catheter-related infections by using maximal sterile barrier precautions during insertion. *Infect Control Hosp Epidemiol* 1994;**15**:231–8.
8. Maki DG, Ringer M, Alvarado CJ. Prospective randomised trial of povidone–iodine, alcohol, and chlorhexidine for prevention of infection associated with central venous and arterial catheters. *Lancet* 1991;**338**:339–43.
9. Humar A, Ostromecki A, Direnfield J, *et al.* Prosepective randomised trial of 10% povidone–iodine versus 0·5% tincture of chlorhexidine as cutaneous antisepsis for prevention of central venous catheter infection. *Clin Infect Dis* 2000;**31**:1001–7.
10. Eggiman P, Harbarth S, Constatin M, Touveneau S, Chevrolet J, Pittet D. Impact of a prevention strategy targeted at vascular-access care on incidence of infections acquired in intensive care. *Lancet* 2000;**355**:1864–8.
11. Maki DG, Stolz SM, Wheeler S, Mermel LA. Prevention of central venous catheter-related bloodstream infection by use of an antiseptic-impregnated catheter: a randomized, controlled trial. *Ann Intern Med* 1997;**127**:257–66.
12. Veenstra DL, Saint S, Saha S, Lumley T, Sullivan SD. Efficacy of antiseptic-impregnated central venous catheters in preventing catheter-related bloodstream infection: a meta-analysis. *JAMA* 1999;**281**:261–7.
13. Veenstra DL, Saint S, Sullivan SD. Cost-effectiveness of antiseptic-impregnated central venous catheters for the prevention of catheter-related bloodstream infection. *JAMA* 1999;**282**:554–60.
14. Walder B, Pittet D, Tramèr M. Prevention of bloodstream infections with central venous catheters treated with anti-infective agents depends on catheter type and insertion time: evidence from a meta-analysis. *Infect Control Hosp Epidemiol* 2002;**23**:748–56.
15. Raad I, Darouiche R, Dupuis J, *et al.* Central venous catheters coated with minocycline and rifampicin for the prevention of catheter-related colonization and bloodstream infections: a randomized, double-blind trial. *Ann Intern Med* 1997;**127**:267–74.
16. Darouiche RO, Issam IR, Heard SO, *et al.* A comparison of two antimicrobial-impregnated central venous catheters. *N Engl J Med* 1999;**340**:1–8.
17. Ruesch S, Walder B, Tramèr T. Complications of central venous catheters: internal jugular versus subclavian access – a systematic review. *Crit Care Med* 2002;**30**:454–60.
18. Merrer J, De Jonghe B, Golliot F, *et al.* Complications of femoral and subclavian venous catheterization in critically ill patients: a randomized controlled trial. *JAMA* 2001;**286**:700–7.
19. Stenzel JP, Green TG, Fuhrman BP, Carlson PE, Marchessault RP. Percutaneous femoral venous catheterizations: a prospective study of complications. *J Pediatr* 1989;**114**:411–5.
20. Randolph AG, Cook DJ, Gonzales CA, Pribble CG. Ultrasound guidance for the placement of central venous catheters: a meta-analysis of the literature. *Crit Care Med* 1996;**24**:2053–8.
21. Keenan SP. Use of ultrasound to place central lines. *J Crit Care* 2002;**17**:126–37.
22. Randolph AG, Cook DJ, Gonzales CA, Brun-Buisson C. Tunneling short-term central venous catheters to prevent catheter-related infection: a meta-analysis of randomized controlled trials. *Crit Care Med* 1998;**26**:1452–7.
23. Raad II, Luna M, Khalil SA, Costerton JW, Lam C, Bodey GP. The relationship between the thrombotic and infectious complications of central venous catheters. *JAMA* 1994;**271**:1014–6.
24. Randolph AG, Cook DJ, Gonzales CA, Andrew M. Benefit of heparin in central venous and pulmonary artery catheters: a meta-analysis of randomised controlled trials. *Chest* 1998;**113**:165–71.
25. Pierce CM, Wade A, Mok Q. Heparin-bonded central venous lines reduced thrombotic and infective complications in critically ill children. *Intensive Care Med* 2000;**26**:967–72.
26. Hoffmann KK, Weber DJ, Samsa GP, Rutala WA. Transparent polyurethane film as an intravenous catheter dressing: a meta-analysis of the infection risks. *JAMA* 1992;**267**:2072–6.

27. Cook DJ, Randolph AG, Kernerman P, *et al*. Central venous catheter replacement strategies: a systematic review of the literature. *Crit Care Med* 1997;**25**:1417–24.
28. Ely EW. Challenges encountered in challenging physicians' practice styles: the ventilator weaning experience. *Intensive Care Med* 1998;**24**:539–41.
29. Bero LA, Grilli R, Grimshaw JM, Harvey E, Oxman AD, Thomson MA. Closing the gap between research and practice: an overview of systematic reviews of interventions to promote the implementation of research findings. The Cochrane Effective Practice and Organisation of Care Review Group. *BMJ* 1998;**317**:465–8.

Part III
Dissemination, implementation, and research agenda

11: The Cochrane Collaboration – what is it about?

TOM PEDERSEN

The Cochrane Collaboration is a major focus of activity, and a rich source of information within the evidence-based medicine movement. The term evidence-based medicine (EBM) originated at McMaster University in Canada, and has been defined as "the conscientious, explicit and judicious use of the best evidence in making decisions about the care of individual patients".[1-3] Thus, to practice EBM is to integrate clinical expertise with the best available external evidence from systematic research. The practice of EBM has been described by Sackett,[3] and the use of EBM in anaesthesia has recently been overviewed by Pronovost et al.,[4] Pedersen and Møller,[5] and Pedersen et al.[6]

Already in 1972, the British epidemiologist Archie Cochrane published his view of the principles on which the delivery of health care should be based.[7] He wrote: "It is surely a great criticism of our profession that we have not organised a critical summary, by speciality or subspeciality, adapted periodically, of all relevant randomised controlled trials". His criticism is still relevant in that people wanting to make well informed decisions about health care are often confronted by hundreds of thousands of potentially relevant research reports. No one can be expected to sift through these mountains of evidence to discover which forms of health care are more likely to do good than harm. Put simply, he stated that limited resources should be used equitably to provide care of proven benefit. Cochrane promoted randomised controlled trials as the most reliable source of evidence on which to base decisions about the effectiveness of healthcare interventions. He advocated the compilation of a comprehensive catalogue of definitive reviews of scientifically valid clinical trials for each speciality. These regularly updated reviews could be consulted to assist with clinical decision making. Medical interventions would thus be scientifically based on properly planned and executed clinical trials (distilled where possible into equally scientifically valid reviews) rather than on anecdote, habit, selective experience, faulty memory, or a skewed sample of the relevant clinical trials, as is often the case. The impact of Cochrane's book *Effectiveness and Efficiency*[7] was not fully recognised at the time, but it captured the essence of today's evidence-based medicine movement. Cochrane's vision of a reliable, comprehensive, and accurate medical database, the Cochrane Library, is approaching reality.

What is the Cochrane Collaboration?

The Cochrane Collaboration is a worldwide organisation. It compromises 50 collaborative review groups (Box 11.1), nine field groups, 10 method groups, 14 Cochrane Centres, and the Cochrane Collaboration Steering Group (Figure 11.1). Collaborative review groups are composed of persons from around the world who share an interest in developing and maintaining systematic reviews relevant to a particular health area. Groups are co-ordinated by an editorial team who edit and assemble completed reviews into modules for inclusion in The Cochrane Library (http://www.update-software.com/cochrane/). The Cochrane Collaboration Steering Group is elected to develop policies and strategies for the Collaboration. It has several subgroups responsible for specific tasks. The Steering Group is supported by the Collaboration Secretariat. Methods Groups are composed of individuals with an interest and expertise in the science of systematic reviews. They provide advice and support to the Collaboration in the development of the methods of systematic reviews. Each review group is supported by a Centre. For example, the anaesthesia group is based in Copenhagen and its supporting centre (the Nordic Cochrane Centre) is based in Copenhagen too. Fields/Networks emerge around areas of interest that extend across a number of health problems. For example, a field co-ordinator in indigenous health care would identify health issues of importance to indigenous populations and facilitate reviews across the relevant review groups in the interests of this population. The work of Collaborative Review Groups, Methods Groups, Fields/Networks, and the Consumer Network is facilitated in a variety of ways by the work of more than a dozen Cochrane Centres around the world. They share responsibility for helping to co-ordinate and support members of the Collaboration in areas such as training, and they promote the objectives of the Collaboration at national level.

The first Cochrane Centre was opened in October 1992 in Oxford, United Kingdom. One year later, the Cochrane Collaboration was founded as a non-profit organisation. It was established as a company, limited by guarantee, and registered as a charity in the United Kingdom. The first Cochrane systematic reviews were prepared by the Pregnancy and Childbirth Group. These reviews have had considerable influence on obstetric and paediatric practice

Box 11.1 All Collaborative Review Groups 2002

- **Acute Respiratory Infections Group:**
  http://www.cochrane.org/cochrane/regcrgs.htm#1750
- **Airways Group:** http://www.cochrane.org/cochrane/regcrgs.htm#1747
- **Anaesthesia Group:**
  http://www.cochrane.org/cochrane/regcrgs.htm#ANA
- **Back Group:** http://www.cochrane.org/cochrane/regcrgs.htm#1973
- **Breast Cancer Group:**
  http://www.cochrane.org/cochrane/regcrgs.htm#1780
- **Colorectal Cancer Group:**
  http://www.cochrane.org/cochrane/regcrgs.htm#3448
- **Consumers and Communication Group:**
  http://www.cochrane.org/cochrane/regcrgs.htm#1769
- **Cystic Fibrosis and Genetic Disorders Group:**
  http://www.cochrane.org/cochrane/regcrgs.htm#1764
- **Dementia and Cognitive Improvement Group:**
  http://www.cochrane.org/cochrane/regcrgs.htm#1759
- **Depression, Anxiety and Neurosis Group:**
  http://www.cochrane.org/cochrane/regcrgs.htm#1776
- **Developmental, Psychosocial and Learning Problems Group:**
  http://www.cochrane.org/cochrane/regcrgs.htm#1980
- **Drug and Alcohol Group:**
  http://www.cochrane.org/cochrane/regcrgs.htm#2866
- **Ear, Nose and Throat Disorders Group:**
  http://www.cochrane.org/cochrane/regcrgs.htm#4194
- **Effective Practice and Organisation of Care Group:**
  http://www.cochrane.org/cochrane/regcrgs.htm#1755
- **Epilepsy Group:** http://www.cochrane.org/cochrane/regcrgs.htm#1766
- **Eyes and Vision Group:**
  http://www.cochrane.org/cochrane/regcrgs.htm#1777
- **Fertility Regulation Group:**
  http://www.cochrane.org/cochrane/regcrgs.htm#1985
- **Gynaecological Cancer Group:**
  http://www.cochrane.org/cochrane/regcrgs.htm#1978
- **Haematological Malignancies Group:**
  http://www.cochrane.org/cochrane/regcrgs.htm#LHG
- **Heart Group:** http://www.cochrane.org/cochrane/regcrgs.htm#3805
- **Hepato-Biliary Group:**
  http://www.cochrane.org/cochrane/regcrgs.htm#1977
- **HIV/AIDS Group:** http://www.cochrane.org/cochrane/regcrgs.htm#1775
- **Hypertension Group:**
  http://www.cochrane.org/cochrane/regcrgs.htm#1778
- **Incontinence Group (website):** http://www.otago.ac.nz/cure/
- **Infectious Diseases Group:**
  http://www.cochrane.org/cochrane/regcrgs.htm#1757
- **Inflammatory Bowel Disease Group:**
  http://www.cochrane.org/cochrane/regcrgs.htm#1758
- **Injuries Group:** http://www.cochrane.org/cochrane/regcrgs.htm#1774
- **Lung Cancer Group:**
  http://www.cochrane.org/cochrane/regcrgs.htm#3806
- **Menstrual Disorders and Subfertility Group:**
  http://www.cochrane.org/cochrane/regcrgs.htm#1763

(Continued)

Box 11.1 *(Continued)*

- **Metabolic and Endocrine Disorders Group:**
  http://www.cochrane.org/cochrane/regcrgs.htm#MAED
- **Movement Disorders Group:**
  http://www.cochrane.org/cochrane/regcrgs.htm#2016
- **Multiple Sclerosis Group:**
  http://www.cochrane.org/cochrane/regcrgs.htm#2993
- **Musculoskeletal Group:**
  http://www.cochrane.org/cochrane/regcrgs.htm#1760
- **Musculoskeletal Injuries:**
  http://www.cochrane.org/cochrane/regcrgs.htm#1752
- **Neonatal Group:** http://www.cochrane.org/cochrane/regcrgs.htm#1782
- **Neuromuscular Disease Group:**
  http://www.cochrane.org/cochrane/regcrgs.htm#3802
- **Oral Health Group:**
  http://www.cochrane.org/cochrane/regcrgs.htm#1754
- **Pain, Palliative Care and Supportive Care:**
  http://www.cochrane.org/cochrane/regcrgs.htm#2966
- **Peripheral Vascular Diseases Group:**
  http://www.cochrane.org/cochrane/regcrgs.htm#1748
- **Pregnancy and Childbirth Group:**
  http://www.cochrane.org/cochrane/regcrgs.htm#1765
- **Prostatic Diseases and Urologic Cancers Group:**
  http://www.cochrane.org/cochrane/regcrgs.htm#1781
- **Renal Group:** http://www.cochrane.org/cochrane/regcrgs.htm#1979
- **Schizophrenia Group:**
  http://www.cochrane.org/cochrane/regcrgs.htm#1762
- **Sexually Transmitted Diseases Group:**
  http://www.cochrane.org/cochrane/regcrgs.htm#3799
- **Skin Group:** http://www.cochrane.org/cochrane/regcrgs.htm#1982
- **Stroke Group:** http://www.cochrane.org/cochrane/regcrgs.htm#1749
- **Subfertility Group:** see Menstrual Disorders
- **Tobacco Addiction Group:**
  http://www.cochrane.org/cochrane/regcrgs.htm#1761
- **Upper Gastrointestinal & Pancreatic Diseases Group:**
  http://www.cochrane.org/cochrane/regcrgs.htm#1981
- **Wounds Group:** http://www.cochrane.org/cochrane/regcrgs.htm#1753

---

throughout the world. This has resulted in increased interest from health professionals and government organisations in expanding the scope to other areas of health care. The Cochrane Collaboration's work today is based on 10 key principles (Box 11.2).

An important contribution of the Cochrane Collaboration is the identification of controlled studies and the creation of a specialised register. This register houses the identified trials that can be accessed for conducting systematic reviews. The reviews prepared within the Collaboration are published in The Cochrane Database of Systematic Reviews, and can be revised and updated every three months if

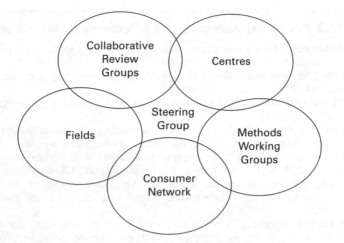

Figure 11.1 The structure of the Cochrane Collaboration

necessary. All outcomes from the Cochrane Collaboration are published electronically on CD Rom and via the internet. The Cochrane Library gives information on ongoing and completed Cochrane reviews. It provides a database of other identified completed reviews, a register of bibliographic information on over 250 000 controlled trials and information about the Cochrane Review Groups. The Cochrane Library is widely acknowledged as the best single source of evidence about the effects of healthcare interventions. It contains The Cochrane Controlled Trials Register, which is now recognised as the most comprehensive bibliography of published reports of controlled trials available.

Collaborative Review Groups

The main work of the Cochrane Collaboration is performed by the Collaborative Review Groups. These are responsible for the preparation and maintenance of Cochrane reviews. A Collaborative Review Group consists of individuals from around the world who share an interest in a particular health topic. Collaborative Review Groups are co-ordinated by an editorial team comprising a Co-ordinating Editor, several other editors, and the Group Co-ordinator. Other members of the Groups include reviewers (who write and update the systematic reviews), peer referees (individuals not involved with systematic review who offer editorial suggestions before publication), hand-searchers (who search for randomised controlled

---

Box 11.2 The 10 key principles of the Cochrane Collaboration

- **Collaborating,** by internally and externally fostering good communications, open decision making, and team work
- **Building on the enthusiasm of individuals,** by involving and supporting people of different skills and background
- **Avoiding duplication,** by good management and co-ordination to maximise economy of effort
- **Minimising bias,** through a variety of approaches such as scientific rigour, ensuring broad participation, and avoiding conflicts of interest
- **Keeping up to date,** by a commitment to ensure that Cochrane reviews are maintained through identification and incorporation of new evidence
- **Striving for relevance,** by promoting the assessment of healthcare interventions using outcomes that matter to people making choices in health care
- **Promoting access,** by wide dissemination of the outputs of the Collaboration, taking advantage of strategic alliances, and by promoting appropriate prices, content, and media to meet the needs of users worldwide
- **Ensuring quality,** by being open and responsive to criticism, applying advances in methodology, developing systems for quality improvement
- **Continuity,** by ensuring that responsibility for reviews, editorial processes, and key functions is maintained and renewed
- **Enabling wide participation** in the work of the Collaboration by reducing barriers to contributing and by encouraging diversity

trials in journals), consumers (people using the prevention or health services), and other interested parties. The primary task of a Collaborative Review Group is to conduct and regularly update systematic reviews of prevention and healthcare issues within the scope of its group. Each Collaborative Review Group creates a specialised register of methodologically sound controlled studies that are relevant to their group. The register is meant to contain both published and unpublished studies, and studies in all languages to avoid publication bias.[8]

The Cochrane Anaesthesia Review Group

The idea of forming the Cochrane Anaesthesia Review Group arose in 1997. The Cochrane Anaesthesia Review Group was established in February 2000 in Copenhagen. The main goal of the Cochrane Anaesthesia Review Group is to conduct systematic reviews of randomised controlled trials and other controlled clinical trials of interventions.[5,6] The scope covers anaesthesia, peri-operative medicine, intensive care medicine, resuscitation, and emergency medicine.

The editorial process

A review is initially registered with a Cochrane Review Group as a title. That title will become a protocol, which prospectively sets out what is being tested, why, and how it will be done. The complete systematic review adheres to the protocol in order to maintain uniformity and minimise bias. Systematic reviews performed by the Cochrane Anaesthesia Review Group are reviews of studies in which evidence has been systematically searched for, studied, assessed, and summarised according to predetermined criteria.

Titles

To register a title with the Cochrane Anaesthesia Review Group, a reviewer submits a registration form (available on the Cochrane Anaesthesia Review Group's website: http://www.carg.dk, or on request from the editorial office). The registration form should include contact details for the reviewers, a preliminary title, and a synopsis describing the background, participants, interventions, outcomes, and keywords. After the title has been approved by the Co-ordinating Editors, and the Review Group Co-ordinator has excluded any potential duplication of work or conflicts of interest with other Cochrane groups, the title is registered. The reviewer is then sent guidelines for writing a systematic review ("Tips for reviewers"); he or she is advised to download and read the Cochrane Reviewer's Handbook (http://www.cochrane.org/cochrane/hbook.htm) and glossary, and is sent details of Cochrane training workshops.

Protocols and reviews

Protocols and reviews are prepared using the Cochrane Collaboration's Review Manager software, RevMan (which is available on CD Rom from the editorial office or can be downloaded from http://www.cochrane.org/cochrane/revman.htm). Reviewers who do not have the computer capability to access RevMan should contact the editorial office. The Review Group Co-ordinator acknowledges receipt of the protocol in the editorial office and forwards the protocol, along with guidelines for editing (see http://www.carg.dk: "Tips for editors/peer referees") to the assigned Cochrane Anaesthesia Review Group editor and two peer referees. The editor and peer referees evaluate and comment on the review title, background, objectives, selection criteria, search strategy, methodology, and the language of the protocol. The protocol – and later, the systematic review (the principal output of the Collaboration) – will be published electronically in successive issues of The Cochrane Library's Database of Systematic Reviews.

Updating

Reviewers are expected to include new trials and to update their reviews annually, or in response to criticism from readers that is published electronically in the Cochrane Library. The editorial office will provide each reviewer with additional annual references within the scope of the review from the specialised register. The same Cochrane Anaesthesia Review Group Editor who evaluated the protocol and its resulting review will edit the updated review in the same manner. Reviews that remain unrevised for more than two years will be flagged automatically on the Cochrane Library. If the reviewer does not update the review, it may be re-allocated or withdrawn.

Specialised Register (SR-ANAESTH)

The Cochrane Anaesthesia Review Group maintains a register of more than 25 000 randomised controlled trials and controlled clinical trials related to anaesthesia, perioperative medicine, intensive care medicine, pre-hospital medicine, resuscitation, and emergency medicine. The register is maintained on ProCite software, and searches for trials are executed quarterly. Trials included in the register are tagged SR-ANAESTH, and the tag term may be searched in the Cochrane Library. Access to the register is available to reviewers and other members of the Cochrane Anaesthesia Review Group.

Consumer representation

One of the goals of the Cochrane Collaboration is to make Cochrane evidence accessible to consumers through the Cochrane Library. The Cochrane Anaesthesia Review Group is liaising with other Review Consumer Groups in order to set up good communications and to learn how to successfully involve in our group the public who are undergoing anaesthesia care. At present, the Cochrane Anaesthesia Review Group has only a few consumers but we are in the process of collaborating with other consumer groups. More information is given on The Cochrane Consumers Network's website (www.cochraneconsumer.com).

Conclusion

The importance of the Cochrane Collaboration and evidence-based medicine has become widely recognised by health professionals and lay people alike. Progress in applying these principles to anaesthesia and perioperative and intensive medicine, as illustrated by Pronovost et al.[4] and Wijetunge and Baldock,[9] has been slow for a variety of reasons. Firstly, hard evidence to support many treatments is simply not available because properly designed studies have not been performed. Secondly, the evidence may exist, but it may not be easily accessible to those making the decisions. Thirdly, even when available, the evidence may not be accepted by those delivering care, particularly if it seems to be in conflict with perceived wisdom or personal experience or if it threatens a vested interest. However, the vision statement of the Cochrane Collaboration in the future is: *Healthcare decision making throughout the world will be informed by high quality, timely research evidence, and the Cochrane Collaboration will play a pivotal role in the production and dissemination of this evidence across all areas of health care.*

References

1. Sackett DL, Rosenberg WM, Gray JA, *et al*. Evidence based medicine: what it is and what it isn't [editorial]. *BMJ* 1996;**312**:71–2.
2. Sackett DL, Richardson WS, Rosenberg WM, *et al*. *Evidence-based medicine. How to practice and teach evidence-based medicine*. Edinburgh: Churchhill Livingstone, 1997.
3. Evidence-Based Medicine Working Group. Evidence-based medicine: a new approach to teaching the practice of medicine. *JAMA* 1992;**268**:2420–5.
4. Pronovost PJ, Berenholtz SM, Dorman T, *et al*. Evidence-based medicine in anesthesiology. *Anesth Analg* 2001;**92**:787–94.
5. Pedersen T, Møller AM. How to use evidence-based medicine in anaesthesiology. *Acta Anaesth Scand* 2001;**45**:267–74.
6. Pedersen T, Møller AM, Cracknell J. The mission of the Cochrane Anaesthesia Review Group: preparing and disseminating systematic reviews of the effect of health care in anesthesiology. *Anesth Analg* 2002;**95**:1012–8.
7. Cochrane A. *Effectiveness and efficiency. Random reflections on health services*. London: Nuffield Provicial Hospitals Trust, 1972.
8. Crombie IK. *Critical appraisal*. London: BMJ Publishing Group, 1999.
9. Wijetunge A, Baldock GJ. Evidence-based intensive care medicine [editorial]. *Anaesthesia* 1998;**53**:419–21.

12: Cost effectiveness of anaesthesia and analgesia

CERI J PHILLIPS

"I even believe that being efficient is a moral obligation, not just a managerial convenience, for not to be efficient means imposing avoidable death and unnecessary suffering on people who might have benefited from the resources which are being used wastefully."

Alan Williams[1]

Introduction

The management of pain represents a major clinical, social, and economic problem. The advent of modern anaesthetics and analgesics has ameliorated its effects, but even in hospital settings in recent years, nearly nine out of every 10 patients have experienced pain levels considered to be excessive.[2,3] This proportion represents a major challenge to those involved in the provision of services. This book has shown the increase in evidence in anaesthesia and analgesia, and although the debate surrounding the relevance and role of evidence-based health care continues,[4-9] it is now recognised that the combination of clinical expertise, current best evidence, and patient ownership of treatment regimens should result in the provision of effective treatments.[10,11] However, in all areas of health care there are other factors that need to inform decisions regarding service provision and resource allocation. The aim of this chapter is to explore the role of economic evaluation and the notion of equity alongside the assessment of evidence in decisions relating to resource allocation and service provision in anaesthesia and analgesia.

Economics and evidence-based anaesthesia and analgesia

The economic problem arises because there will never be enough resources to completely satisfy human desires. Because resources are scarce, choices have to be made about different ways of using them.

When resources are used in one way, they are not available for use in other activities and the benefits that would have resulted are sacrificed. These sacrifices are referred to as "opportunity cost" and, in this sense, cost is the value placed on the sacrifices, regardless of whether or not money is paid for them.

The economic problem is a major issue for virtually all healthcare systems, confronted as they are by an exponential increase in demand for healthcare services against a background of limited resources with which to meet these levels of demand. In addition, despite the growth in evidence relating to effectiveness and ineffectiveness, there remain many areas in which there is a dearth of such evidence.

Economic evaluation and anaesthesia and analgesia

Economic evaluation is based on the notion of *efficiency*. Trials and systematic reviews provide evidence relating to the relative efficacy and effectiveness of interventions,* but this alone does not address the issue of whether scarce resources are being used in the most beneficial way. Efficiency considers both the costs and the benefits and the relationship between them. However, there are very few examples of good quality cost information being available to use alongside evidence on effectiveness. The costs of interventions and programmes are often constructed on the basis of prices and fees paid, rather than on any notion of opportunity cost. Studies tend to adopt a narrow perspective based on health service budgets, rather than on a broader societal perspective, where all changes in resource utilisation are taken into account, regardless of which budget or which aspect of society is affected.[12] However, despite these limitations, the case for undertaking economic evaluations alongside systematic reviews is strong as they provide a "consideration of the resource consequences of alternative interventions" and "methods for valuing health (and other) outcomes", especially when "significant amounts of health care resources are at stake and when trade-offs between costs and outcomes, or between different types of outcomes are likely".[13] Figure 12.1 illustrates the healthcare dilemma.

The basic framework of economic evaluation in health care is shown in Figure 12.2 below. It involves a comparison of the costs involved and the benefits derived from each of the alternative interventions or programmes (which may include doing nothing).[14]

---

*For definitions of these concepts see Currie G, Manns B. Glossary of terms for health economics and systematic review. In: Donaldson C, *et al. Evidence-based health economics*. London: BMJ Books, 2002.

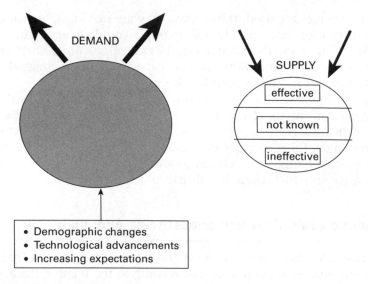

Figure 12.1 The healthcare dilemma

In assessing the costs (inputs) and benefits (outputs and outcomes), three stages can be distinguished – identification, measurement, and valuation.

Identification of costs and benefits

The identification of costs and benefits involves placing them in certain categories.

Categories of costs

Types of cost:

- *Direct costs*: these relate to the use of resources directly as a result of the anaesthetic process. They include drug acquisition costs, cost of staff time involved in delivering and administering the procedures, costs of materials and equipment plus costs to organisations involved in the process and to patients, in terms of transport costs and out-of-pocket expenses.
- *Indirect costs*: these relate to losses to society incurred – for example, as a result of the impact of postoperative pain or nausea and vomiting on production, domestic responsibilities, and social and leisure activities.
- *Intangibles*: these relate to the distress, suffering, anxiety, and impact on quality of life resulting from, for example, postoperative infections and other complications.

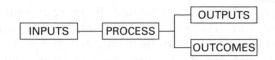

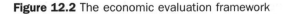

Figure 12.2 The economic evaluation framework

Categories of effects/benefits

Types of effect/benefit:

- *Disease-specific effects*: specific outputs and outcomes resulting from anaesthesia, such as recovery time, improvements in pain scores, and return to normal functioning.
- *Mortality and survival*: changes in life expectancy that may result from the intervention, and measures such as life years saved and lives saved.
- *Utility effects*: measures that can be used to compare health status across all healthcare interventions, such as healthy days and quality adjusted life years (QALYs).
- *Economic effects*: resources released, and expressed in monetary terms, by improvement in recovery and discharge times and the treatment of emesis rather than prophylaxis.

Economic evaluation is not a costless exercise, and principles sometimes need to be compromised in the interests of practicality. Although it may be desirable to identify all costs and benefits, in practice some are likely to be trivial and not worth collecting. In addition, evidence relating to costs is unlikely to be present in one single source, and information may have to be collected from databases, administrative records, case records, clinical trials, systematic reviews, and observational studies. The quality of such evidence is variable and it is essential that the validity of assumptions and the impact of changes in costs and benefits are assessed in a sensitivity analysis as part of the economic evaluation.

Measurement of costs and benefits

In deciding which costs and benefits to measure it is usual to isolate those that are important and whose exclusion would bias the result of the evaluation. For those remaining, an assessment is made of the additional value given to the evaluation relative to the extra cost of collecting. Anything that is expensive to collect but whose inclusion is unlikely to influence the overall result need not be measured.

Costs and benefits are initially measured in relevant physical units such as hours of staff time, quantity of medication, equipment usage, and number of patients being treated. If the economic evaluation is being carried out alongside a randomised controlled trial the resources that are required can be monitored prospectively. However, when it is carried out in conjunction with a systematic review it becomes more difficult, because costs are specific to a particular setting and country, and the studies are likely to have been undertaken in different settings and across many countries.

Care has to be taken when measuring benefits because trials have limited time-scales, and follow-up periods may not resemble disease progression and patient management pathways. For example, the use of non-steroidal anti-inflammatory drugs (NSAIDs) over a period of time has been shown to cause significant upper gastrointestinal side effects, which may lead to hospitalisation, surgery or even death. This could lead to significant iatrogenic costs being incurred,[15-19] which would not be picked up by a narrow time-constrained analysis of cost effectiveness.

In measuring costs and benefits it is important to distinguish between marginal and average costs and benefits. Average cost is the total cost divided by the number of units, whereas marginal cost is the cost of generating one additional unit. Differences between them can be considerable and marginal costs can change dramatically. For example, in the management of postoperative nausea and vomiting (PONV), the additional cost of one additional patient who experiences no more than one episode of PONV when treatment is switched from 1 mg of ondansetron to 4 mg amounted to an additional 60 mg of drug, whereas the cost of one additional PONV-free patient after switching prophylaxis from 4 mg to 8 mg amounted to over 900 mg in low-risk groups and over 1800 mg in high-risk groups.[20]

Another consideration is that average cost may not be an accurate reflection of reality. For example, the average cost of a hospital episode includes the relatively high levels of resource utilisation during the first few days and the lower hotel costs during the latter stages. Therefore, the issue of whether to measure cost in terms of marginal or average depends very much on the nature of the comparison and policy setting.[12] For example, in a comparison of two anaesthetic programmes that require different types of infrastructure, average costs are recommended because the fixed costs element would be ignored by the use of marginal cost. However, when the choice is between two or more analgesics the use of marginal cost rather than average would be more appropriate.

There is also debate as to whether the human capital approach (where a year of working time lost is measured by average salary) or the friction method (where production losses are dealt with by transferring work lost to other workers) should be used in measuring indirect costs. The differences in results may be highly significant. For example, the indirect non-medical cost of neck pain in the Netherlands in 1996 was estimated at US$ 526·5 million using the human capital approach and US$ 96·3 million using the friction cost method.[21]

Quantifying health effects may also create difficulties. Outcome measures from clinical trials and systematic reviews are widely used in cost-effectiveness analysis, but to assess whether resources would generate additional benefits if used elsewhere, a form of *common currency* needs to be used. For example, would it be more efficient to use more effective, but more expensive, epidural patient-controlled analgesia after caesarean section rather than intrathecal morphine,[22] or use the same resources to help finance an acute pain service?[23] Specific measures are not helpful in this context. Attention has been focused on measures to assess the impact of interventions on health related quality of life, as well as life expectancy. There are several approaches, which combine these two attributes into a single measure of health status. One of the most common is that of the quality adjusted life year (QALY), which assigns a score corresponding to the health related quality of life during a particular time period. Therefore, if a programme results in an additional 10 years of life, but each of the additional life years will be of less than perfect health – for example, 0·75 on a 0–1 scale, where 0 represents death* and 1 represents perfect health – then the programme will have resulted in 7·5 QALYs.

It is important that the approach used to measure costs and benefits is made explicit and that appropriate time scales are employed so that decision makers are aware of all relevant costs and benefits. Increasing reliance is being placed on modelling to simulate a patient's or a population's life experience under a variety of intervention scenarios, and although contentious, they show how cost-effectiveness ratios might change if the values of key parameters are adjusted.

Valuation of costs and benefits

The extent to which a value needs to be put on the benefits generated depends on the type of appraisal. In cost-effectiveness analysis the outcomes are simply counted. In cost–utility analysis the outcomes are expressed in terms of a health status measure such as QALYs. Cost–benefit analysis, however, requires that benefits are valued in monetary terms, so that the value of costs and benefits can be compared directly. When market valuations exist they can be used as a method for valuing benefits (as long as they have been adjusted to exclude taxation and subsidies), whereas the compensation paid by a court to offset damages resulting from medical negligence could also be used. The main difficulty arises when trying to place a monetary value on intangibles, where market prices do not exist. There are two main techniques that

---

*It is possible to have negative states of health that are worse than death.

can be used here – *conjoint analysis*[24] and *willingness-to-pay*.[25] Conjoint analysis assumes that the attributes of a service determine the satisfaction (utility) that individuals receive from that service, whereas willingness-to-pay is based on the premise that the maximum amount of money an individual is willing to pay for a commodity is an indicator of the value to them of that commodity. For example, in one study the median willingness-to-pay for a reduction to reduce the risk of PONV from a 1-in-3 chance to a 1-in-10 chance was £50.[26]

It is important that all costs and benefits are included in the "cost–benefit" balance sheet, irrespective of whether they are measured or valued, so that decision makers are fully aware of the consequences of implementing a programme or switching to an alternative intervention.

The process of calculating the cost-effectiveness ratio should take into account the context of the decision. If a new treatment is being considered it is unlikely that it will replace all existing therapies. Instead, some patients are switched to the new treatment, whereas others will remain on existing treatments. In comparing new therapies with placebo or existing alternatives, the question is whether the additional costs of the new therapy justify the additional benefits to be gained. The *incremental cost-effectiveness ratio* (ICER) (difference in costs divided by the difference in benefits) is used to address this issue. The ICER can be placed on a cost-effectiveness plane,[27] as shown in Figure 12.3.

Interventions with ICERs in the north-east quadrant require some consideration. They improve health but cost more than the alternative(s). The decision whether or not to choose them should be based on the level of additional resources available, or by viewing the ICER in the light of a specific acceptable threshold.[27] For example, interventions with cost–QALY ratios of between £3000 and £20 000 are adjudged to be cost-effective when there is evidence of their effectiveness.[28]

Dealing with time and uncertainty: discounting and sensitivity analysis

Most people prefer to delay costs as long as possible and receive benefits as soon as possible. Therefore, costs and benefits that occur today are valued more highly than those that occur in the future, and the current value of any cost or benefit is lower the further in the future that it arises. To allow for this, future costs and benefits are subjected to *discounting*.* There is ongoing debate as to whether non-financial gains

*The approach is quite simple using the formula: $PV = K*(1/(1 + r)^n)$ where PV = present value, K = the nominal value of the cost or benefit, r = the discount rate and n = how many years in the future the cost or benefit arises. If we expect to receive a benefit of £10 000 in five years' time, the present value, based on a discount rate of 5%, is equivalent to £7835.

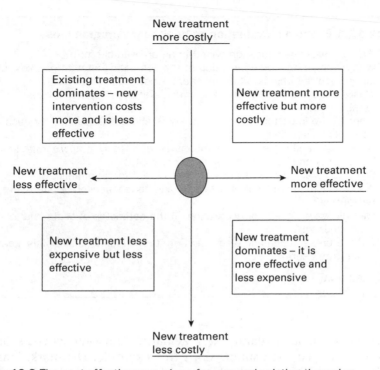

Figure 12.3 The cost-effectiveness plane for new and existing therapies. Adapted from[26]

should be discounted and the current recommendation is that benefits are presented as discounted in the base-case analysis and with no discounting in the sensitivity analysis.[29]

At this stage of the chapter it should be evident that economic evaluation is not an exact science and that findings from such studies should be treated with caution. It is essential when undertaking an economic evaluation that a sensitivity analysis is included. The approach is to test how sensitive are the results obtained by considering "what if"-type scenarios and questions. In other words, the effects of changes in costs and benefits and the discount rate will all have to be assessed before the results of the evaluation can be delivered to the relevant decision maker(s).

Requirements for health economic evaluations

The growth in the number of health economic evaluations has led to the development of guidelines for the conduct, design, and methodology of such studies. A number of countries have made submission of economic evaluations an official requirement for placement of medication on their national formulary (for example,

---

Box 12.1 Economic evaluation of healthcare programmes

- Was a well-defined question posed in an answerable form?
- Was a comprehensive description of the competing alternative given (that is, can you tell who did what, to whom, where, and how often)?
- Was there evidence that the programme's effectiveness had been established?
- Were all the important and relevant costs and consequences for each alternative identified?
- Were costs and consequences measured accurately in appropriate units?
- Were costs and consequences valued credibly?
- Were costs and consequences adjusted for differential timing?
- Was an incremental analysis of costs and consequences of alternatives performed?
- Was allowance made for uncertainty in the estimates of costs and consequences?
- Did the presentation and discussion of study results include all issues of concern to users?

Adapted from[14]

Australia, Canada, Finland, New Zealand, Norway) whereas others have encouraged such submissions (for example, Denmark, France). In the United Kingdom, the National Institute of Clinical Excellence (NICE) expects companies to submit a dossier of evidence of clinical and cost effectiveness relating to their product when an assessment of that particular technology is being undertaken. An example of guidelines is shown in Box 12.1.

Equity considerations in decision making in anaesthesia and analgesia

Concern about persisting and widening health inequalities within and across countries has elevated equity to a high rank among health policy objectives. The aim of reducing health inequalities appears uncontroversial, but there is no consensus on how to deal with policies that may improve efficiency while increasing inequalities or policies that improve fairness while decreasing efficiency.[30] To illustrate, NICE was launched in the United Kingdom on the back of disapproval of the "postcode-prescribing" lottery, which had existed as different health authorities formulated different policies on which treatments they would fund. NICE has been expressly concerned with identifying clinically effective and cost-effective technologies "to remove unfairness in the availability of technologies in different localities and to minimise the possibility of further examples of unfairness or inequity being introduced."[31] However, the implementation of NICE recommendations may not necessarily result in either an improvement in efficiency or a removal of inequities in access and provision.[32-34] Without additional funding, the National Health Service (NHS) at a local level may have to deny funding to other services in order to finance NICE recommendations, as it is a requirement that new treatments approved by NICE have to be funded within three months of the decision.[35] This results in achieving greater equity in some areas of service provision at the expense of creating inequities in others.

The lack of equity in service provision in the UK was highlighted by the Audit Commission, who reported considerable regional variation in the number of hospitals with multidisciplinary teams in acute pain, ranging from just over 40% in some areas to over 70% in others.[2] Similarly, a survey of 105 hospitals from 17 European countries showed that 34% of hospitals had an organised acute pain service, very few hospitals used quality assurance measures, and over 50% of anaesthesiologists were dissatisfied with postoperative pain management on surgical wards.[36]

Evidence and cost effectiveness and their relevance in informing decision making in anaesthesia and analgesia

Deciding which services and treatments should be provided is highly complex and involves a number of different, often conflicting, factors. Information relating to the effectiveness, efficiency, and equity of interventions and programmes needs to be utilised to enhance the quality of the commissioning process and ensure that the best care is provided within available resources. Anaesthesia and analgesia is one area in particular where a system based on joined-up thinking is required.[37] The advent of modern anaesthetics and analgesics and the implementation of evidence-based health care has meant that the effects of pain can be ameliorated to some extent. However, there remain many examples of inefficiencies. Patients suffer unnecessary levels of pain,[2,3] adverse events are estimated to cost the NHS about £500 million a year in additional days spent in hospital,[38] and adverse drug reactions in English hospitals cost £380 million per year, which is equivalent to 15-20 400-bed hospitals.[39] The cost of hospital-acquired infection in England has been estimated at £930 million per annum, with infected patients staying in hospital for two weeks longer than those without infection.[40] It has also been estimated that 5% of the 8.5 million patients admitted to hospitals in England and Wales each year experience preventable adverse events, leading to an additional three million bed days at a cost to the NHS of £1billion a year.[41] Adverse events occurred in 17% of hospital admissions in Australia, half of which were considered preventable and which cost Australian $4.7 billion a year.[42] In the United States, 4% of hospital admissions led to adverse

161

events, resulting in permanent disability in 7% and contributing to death in 14% of cases,[43,44] while in the United Kingdom one-third of adverse events led to at least moderate disability or death.[39]

These data emphasise the sentiment at the beginning of this chapter that when resources are not used efficiently, unnecessary suffering and death result. Appeals for improvements in the quality of postoperative pain management and suggestions offered as to what can be done to remedy the problems and improve the quality of care have been heard in this book (Chapter 4) and elsewhere.[45–48] However, the problem with many healthcare systems is that they are fragmented and narrowly focused, with excessive significance attached to financial budgets,[49] with drug costs often targeted for cutbacks, since they are easy to measure, while other major costs and sources of waste are ignored.[50–53] However, the cost of treatment is not simply the cost of drugs or medical and nursing time but includes recovery times, incidence of side effects, rate of delayed discharge, use of resources in postanaesthesia care and the cost of system deficiencies and problems.[54–57] For example, in a trial to assess the cost effectiveness of interventions for treating pain after limb injury, the unit cost of intravenous ketorolac was three times that of morphine, but the overall cost of morphine was over five times that of ketorolac, with much of the difference accounted for by the management of adverse events.[58]

The adoption of a broader agenda in anaesthesia and analgesia would mean that one of the major objectives underlying decisions was to avoid pain from becoming chronic. Although pain affects everyone to varying degrees, for some it is a permanent feature of their lives and has a profound impact on their quality of life. Also, the economic impact of pain is substantial[59,60] and imposes a greater burden than many other diseases.[59,61]

Therefore, additional work is needed to develop a broader, strategic agenda. Firstly, although the establishment of acute pain services has been associated with significant decreases in postoperative pain scores[61] and improvements in patient satisfaction,[22] these need to be translated into an improvement in recovery times and return to normal functioning in order that their cost-effectiveness can be assessed. Secondly, there have also been calls for cost-effectiveness, cost–utility, and cost–benefit analyses to "determine the appropriate clinical and cost circumstances for the use of patient-controlled analgesia."[62] Thirdly, assessment of the cost-effectiveness of strategies for dealing with PONV are constrained by differences in the outcomes resulting from prophylaxis and treatment. The extent of cost differences between treatment and prophylaxis is large.[19] Therefore, consideration needs to be given to the nature, magnitude, and value attached to such differences and to further work is required to identify what sort of compensation patients might be prepared to "accept" in return for the potential reduction in satisfaction with their care.

These issues highlight the need for a change in approach from all involved in the decision-making process. It has been argued that "... it is not enough to be a good doctor in contemporary anaesthesiology practice ... rather, we must understand economics and business ...".[64] However, it is also necessary that managers understand the professionals' agendas and that policy makers take account of the patients' perspectives and views.

There are signs that attention is being focused on efficiency issues within anaesthetic and analgesic services. A study to move the agenda forward on the cost of medication in acute postoperative pain has provided useful data relating to the cost and practice of medicines management.[65] Other studies have shown that by changing anaesthetic technique and practice, demand on intensive care beds was reduced[66] and throughput in postanaesthesia care units was improved,[67] and others have discussed whether it is more cost effective to employ a treatment strategy or prophylaxis for PONV.[19,55] A recent study to assess the analgesic efficacy, adverse effects, and cost-effectiveness of a needle-free jet-injection system with lidocaine for the insertion of an intravenous cannula showed that it would cost the particular hospital more than $500 000 each year to use the device with lidocaine 2% for all peripheral cannula insertions. The question posed was whether it would be worth spending $11 to achieve an additional patient with minimal pain, and the solution offered was that targeting patients who were most likely to benefit should be the way forward.[68]

Conclusion

Health policy issues are high on political agendas. Technological advancements, developments in medical science, and increasing expectations of communities as to what is available from healthcare providers continue to focus attention on the healthcare dilemma. This chapter has aimed to show how the utilisation of economic techniques alongside evidence-based practice can enhance the quality of decision making in anaesthesia and analgesia. The healthcare dilemma means that choices will always have to be made regarding the level of resources allocated to health care and, within health care, which areas receive a greater share and which areas receive less (Figure 12.1). In making such choices an explicit set of priorities needs to be established and attitudes changed. The evidence base for the effectiveness of interventions and management strategies in anaesthesia and analgesia is continuously being developed. The recognition of the need to generate evidence relating to resource utilisation and the most beneficial utilisation of available resources is encouraging. However, the existence of ineffectiveness and inefficiencies in service provision has to be addressed. The development of evidence-based practice, a

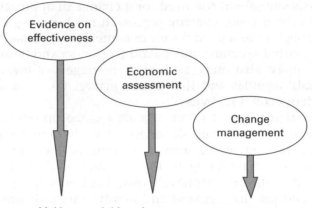

Figure 12.4 Making things happen in the management of pain.
Source: http://www.jr2.ox.ac.uk/bandolier/bandopubs/RAMnhsfu/NHSfutur.html

recognition that resources are finite and choices have to be made, and an awareness of the need for fairness in resource allocation and service provision, are major steps along the road to answering the question of how much additional resources should be put into anaesthetics and pain services and into health care in general. What is left is the will to move along the road of change and make things happen (Figure 12.4).

References

1. Alan Williams. Ethics, clinical freedom and the doctors' role. In: Culyer AJ et al., eds. *Competition in health care: reforming the NHS.* Basingstoke: Macmillan, 1990.
2. Bruster S, Jarman B, Bosanquet N, *et al.* National survey of hospital patients. *BMJ* 1994;**309**:1542–6.
3. *Anaesthesia under examination: the efficiency and effectiveness of anaesthesia and pain relief services in England and Wales.* London: Audit Commission, 1997.
4. Black N. Evidence-based policy: proceed with care. *BMJ* 2001;**323**:275–8.
5. Donald A. Research must be taken seriously. *BMJ* 2001;**323**:278–9.
6. Goodman NW. Evidence-based medicine: cautious before using. In: *Evidence based resource in anaesthesia and analgesia.* Tramèr MR, ed. London: BMJ Books, 2000.
7. Leicester G. The seven enemies of evidence-based policy. *Public Money and Management* 1999;**19**:5–7.
8. Walshe K. Evidence based policy: don't be timid. *BMJ* 2001;**323**:1187.
9. Maynard, A. Evidence-based medicine: cost effectiveness and equity are ignored. *BMJ* 1996;**313**:170.
10. Greenhalgh T. Is my practice evidence based? *BMJ* 1996;**313**:957–8.
11. Sackett DL, Rosenberg WMC, Gray JAM, *et al.* Evidence based medicine: what it is and what it isn't. *BMJ* 1996;**312**:71–2.
12. Brouwer W, Rutten F, Koopmanschap M. Costing in economic evaluation. In: Drummond MF, McGuire A, eds. *Economic evaluation in health care: merging theory with practice.* Oxford: Oxford University Press, 2001.
13. Donaldson C, Mugford M, Vale L. Using systematic reviews in economic evaluation: the basic principles. In: Donaldson C, Mugford M, Vale L, eds. *Evidence-based*

health economics: from effectiveness to efficiency in systematic review. London: BMJ Books, 2002.

14. Drummond MF, O'Brien B, Stoddart GL, *et al. Methods for the economic evaluation of healthcare programmes.* Oxford: Oxford University Press, 1997.

15. Moore RA, Phillips CJ. Cost of NSAID adverse effects to the UK National Health Service. *J Med Econ* 1999;2:45–55.

16. Jonsson B, Haglund U. Economic burden of NSAID-induced gastropathy in Sweden. *Scand J Gastroenterol* 2001;**36**:775–9.

17. Herings RM, Klungel OH. An epidemiological approach to assess the economic burden of NSAID-induced gastrointestinal events in The Netherlands. *Pharmacoeconomics* 2001;**19**:655–65.

18. Rahme E, Joseph L, Kong SX, Watson DJ, Le Lorier J. Cost of prescribed NSAID-related gastrointestinal adverse events in elderly patients. *Br J Clin Pharmacol* 2001;**52**:185–92.

19. Page J, Henry D. Consumption of NSAIDs and the development of congestive heart failure in elderly patients: an underrecognized public health problem. *Arch Intern Med* 2000;**160**:777–84.

20. Tramèr MR, Phillips CJ, Reynolds DJM, *et al.* Cost-effectiveness of ondansetron for postoperative nausea and vomiting. *Anaesthesia* 1999;**54**:226–34.

21. Borghouts JAJ, Koes BW, Vondeling H, Bouter LM. Cost-of-illness of neck pain in The Netherlands in 1996. *Pain* 1999;**80**:629–36.

22. Vercauteren M, Vereecken K, La Malfa M, *et al.* Cost-effectiveness of analgesia after Caesarean section: a comparison of intrathecal morphine and epidural PCA. *Acta Anaesthesiol Scand* 2002;**46**:85–90.

23. Tighe SQ, Bie JA, Nelson RA, Skues MA. The acute pain service: effective or expensive care? *Anaesthesia* 1998;**53**:382–403.

24. Ryan M, Hughes J. Using conjoint analysis to value surgical versus medical management of miscarriage. *Health Econ* 1997;6:261–73.

25. Olsen JA, Donaldson C. Helicopters, hearts and hips: using willingness to pay to set priorities for public sector health care programmes. *Soc Sci Med* 1998;**46**:1–12.

26. Diez LL. Assessing the willingness of parents to pay for reducing postoperative emesis in children. *Pharmacoeconomics* 1998;**13**:589–95.

27. Briggs AH. Handling uncertainty in economic evaluation and presenting the results. In: Drummond MF, McGuire A, eds. *Economic evaluation in health care: merging theory with practice.* Oxford: Oxford University Press, 2001.

28. Stevens A, Colin-Jones D, Gabbay J. Quick and clean: authoritative health technology assessment for local health care contracting. *Health Trends* 1995;**27**:37–42.

29. Johannesson M, Jonsson B, Karlsson G. Outcome measurement in economic evaluation. *Health Econ* 1996;5:279–96

30. Sassi F, Le Grand J, Archard L. Equity versus efficiency: a dilemma for the NHS. *BMJ* 2001;**323**:762–3.

31. National Institute for Clinical Excellence. *Technical guidance for manufacturers and sponsors on making a submission to a technology appraisal.* London: National Institute for Clinical Excellence, 2001.

32. Doyle Y. Equity in the new NHS: hard lessons from implementing a local healthcare policy on donepezil. *BMJ* 2001;**323**:222–4.

33. Burke K. No cash to implement NICE, health authorities tell MPs. *BMJ* 2002;**324**:258.

34. Smith R. The failings of NICE. *BMJ* 2000;**321**:1363–4.

35. Dent THS, Sadler M. From guidance to practice: why NICE is not enough. *BMJ* 2002;**324**:842–5.

36. Rawal N, Allvin R, EuroPain Acute Pain Working Party. Acute pain services in Europe: a 17-nation survey of 105 hospitals. *Eur J Anaesthesiol* 1998;**15**:354–63.

37. Phillips CJ. The real cost of pain management. *Anaesthesia* 2001;**56**:1031–3.

38. *A spoonful of sugar: medicines management in NHS hospitals.* London: Audit Commission, 2001.

39. Wiffen P, Gill M, Edwards J, Moore A. Adverse drug reactions in hospital patients: a systematic review of the prospective and retrospective studies. *Bandolier Extra* 2002 June. www.jr2.ox.ac.uk/bandolier/Extraforbando/ADRPM.pdf (accessed 3 April 2003).

40. Plowman R, Graves N, Griffin M, *et al. Socio-economic burden of hospital acquired infection.* London: Public Health Laboratory Service, 2000.

41. Vincent C, Neale G, Woloshynowych M. Adverse events in British hospitals: preliminary retrospective record review. *BMJ* 2001;**322**:517–9.
42. Wilson RM, Runciman WB, Gibberd RW, *et al*. The quality in Australian health care study. *Med J Aust* 1995;**163**:458–71.
43. Brennan TA, Leape LL, Laird NM, *et al*. Incidence of adverse events and negligence in hospitalised patients. *N Engl J Med* 1991;**324**:370–6.
44. Leape LL, Brennan TA, Laird NM, *et al*. Incidence of adverse events and negligence in hospitalised patients: results of the Harvard medical practice study II. *N Engl J Med* 1991;**324**:377–84.
45. McQuay HJ, Moore A, Justins D. Treating acute pain in hospital. *BMJ* 1997;**314**:131–5.
46. Rawal N, Allvin R. Postoperative pain an unnecessary suffering: a model of emergency pain relief implemented in Orebro. *Lakartidningen* 2001;**98**:1648–54.
47. Salomaki TE, Hokajarvi TM, Ranta P, Alahuhta S. Improving the quality of postoperative pain relief. *Eur J Pain* 2000;**4**:367–72.
48. Wilder-Smith OHG, Möhrle JJ, Martin NC. Acute pain management after surgery or in the emergency room in Switzerland: a comparative survey of Swiss anaesthesiologists and surgeons. *Eur J Pain* 2002;**6**:189–201.
49. Taheri PA, Butz DA, Greenfield LJ. Length of stay has minimal impact on the cost of hospital admission. *J Am Coll Surg* 2000;**191**:123–30.
50. Smith I. Cost considerations in the use of anaesthetic drugs. *Pharmacoeconomics* 2001;**19**:469–81.
51. Phillip BK. Practical cost-effective choices: ambulatory general anesthesia. *J Clin Anesth* 1995;**7**:606–13.
52. Kapur PA. Pharmacy acquisition costs: responsible choices versus overutilization of costly pharmaceuticals. *Anesth Analg* 1994;**78**:617–8.
53. Becker KE Jr, Carrithers J. Practical methods of cost containment in anesthesia and surgery. *J Clin Anesth* 1994;**6**:388–99.
54. Orkin FK. Meaningful cost reduction: penny wise, pound foolish. *Anesthesiology* 1995;**83**:1135–7.
55. Suver J, Arikian SR, Doyle JJ, *et al*. Use of anesthesia selection in controlling surgery costs in an HMO hospital. *Clin Ther* 1995;**17**:561–71.
56. White PF, Watcha MF. Pharmacoeconomics in anaesthesia: what are the issues? *Eur J Anaesthesiol* 2001;**18**(Suppl. 23):10–5.
57. Broadway PJ, Jones JG. A method of costing anaesthetic practice. *Anaesthesia* 1995;**50**:56–63.
58. Rainer TH, Jacobs P, Ng YC, *et al*. Cost effectiveness analysis of intravenous ketorolac and morphine for treating pain after limb injury: double blind randomised controlled trial. *BMJ* 2000;**321**:1–9.
59. Maniadakis N, Gray A. The economic burden of back pain in the UK. *Pain* 2000;**84**: 95–103.
60. Belsey J. Primary care workload in the management of chronic pain: a retrospective cohort study using a GP database to identify resource implications for UK primary care. *J Med Econ* 2002;**5**:39–52.
61. Jonsson E. *Back pain, neck pain*. Swedish Council on Technology Assessment in Health Care Report No. 145. Stockholm, 2000.
62. Werner MU, Søholm L, Rotbøll-Nielsen P, Kehlet H. Does an acute pain service improve postoperative outcome? *Anesth Analg* 2002;**95**:1361–72.
63. Jacox A, Carr DB, Mahrenholz DM, Ferrell BM. Cost considerations in patient-controlled analgesia. *Pharmacoeconomics* 1997;**12**:109–20.
64. Chestnut DH. How do we measure (the cost of) pain relief? *Anesthesiology* 2000;**92**: 643–5.
65. Dalton JA, Carlson J, Lindley C, *et al*. Clinical economics: calculating the cost of acute postoperative pain medication. *J Pain Symp Manag* 2000;**19**:295–308.
66. Park GR, Evans TN, Hutchins J, *et al*. Reducing the demand for admission to intensive care after major abdominal surgery by a change in anaesthetic practice and the use of remifentanil. *Eur J Anaesthesiol* 2000;**17**:111–9.
67. Beaussier M, Decorps A, Tilleul P, *et al*. Desflurane improves the throughput of patients in the PACU: a cost-effectiveness comparison with isoflurane. *Can J Anaesth* 2002;**49**:339–46.
68. Lysakowski C, Dumont L, Tramèr MR, Tassonyi E. A needle-free jet-injection system with lidocaine for peripheral intravenous cannula insertion: a randomised controlled trial with cost-effectiveness analysis. *Anesth Analg* 2003;**96**:215–9.

13: From evidence to implementation

ANNA LEE, TONY GIN

Evidence-based clinical decision making has been increasingly guided by the findings from randomised controlled trials and systematic reviews. However, to implement and apply these results in clinical practice is often difficult. Successful transfer of evidence into practice requires timely dissemination of good evidence by effective interventions. In the clinical anaesthetic setting, the percentage of interventions supported by systematic reviews or randomised controlled trials was 32% (95% confidence interval 24·5–39·5%).[1] This chapter will discuss barriers and strategies in implementing evidence, and methods of applying the evidence from systematic reviews to individual patients.

Implementing research evidence

Not all evidence from research can be implemented into clinical practice because of limited resources in the healthcare system. The anticipated benefits of health improvement must be considered with the cost of overcoming the barriers to getting research into practice. Factors to consider when implementing research evidence are the quality of the evidence, the degree of uncertainty of findings, relevance to the clinical setting, and whether the benefits to patient outweigh any adverse effects.[2] The transfer of evidence into clinical practice is often slow, and patients can be denied the benefits of effective treatment. For example, the routine use of thrombolytic therapy for acute myocardial infarction first appeared in 1987, 14 years after a statistically significant ($P = 0.01$) beneficial effect became evident in a cumulative meta-analysis.[3]

Barriers and strategies

The main steps from evidence to practice are shown in Figure 13.1. Several challenges face the anaesthetist who wishes to use systematic reviews as the primary method of keeping up to date with the best available evidence. These include poor quality systematic reviews and

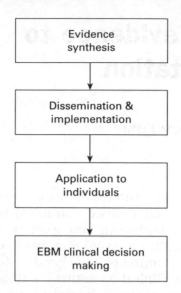

Figure 13.1 Taking steps from evidence to practice in evidence-based medicine (EBM)

the limited number of systematic reviews published in peer reviewed journals on anaesthetics.[4] Over half of all systematic reviews in the anaesthesia literature have major or extensive flaws.[4] Systematic reviews in anaesthesia could be improved by better search strategies to find relevant studies, using methods to avoid selection bias, using validated methods to evaluate the validity of each included study, and assessment of potential sources of bias.[4]

The uptake of research evidence into clinical practice may also improve with the availability of online resources in anaesthesia. These online resources can provide timely and quality information at the point of decision making. Recently, a collaborative link between the Cochrane Anaesthesia Review Group and *Anesthesia and Analgesia* has been developed to disseminate to a wider readership the evidence on interventions in anaesthesia published in the Cochrane Library.[5]

Other barriers to dissemination and timely application of evidence into practice are shown in Box 13.1. Common interventions to promote professional behavioural change include continuing medical education (conferences, courses, workshops, lectures), audit and feedback, clinical practice guidelines, and local consensus processes (physicians agree to the importance of clinical problem and appropriate management treatment).[6] However, some interventions are more effective than others. From the anaesthetist's perspective, most (82%) believe that patients benefit from those anaesthetists who are involved in continuing medical education.[7]

> **Box 13.1 Common barriers to dissemination and timely application of evidence into clinical practice**
>
> - Lack of timely, valid, and relevant information at the point of decision making
> - Lack of time and resources allocated for ongoing training and adaptation of services to apply research findings
> - Lack of high-level critical appraisal skills of clinicians
> - Ignorance of clinicians' beliefs, perceptions, and experience
> - Lack of organisational commitment to change
> - Poor dissemination strategies (for example, didactic lectures, distribution of clinical practice guidelines)
>
> Adapted from [8] and [9]

There is strong evidence that interactive educational meetings are effective in changing physician behaviour and, on occasions, health outcome.[6,10] A randomised controlled trial showed that the use of a computerised advanced cardiac life support (ACLS) simulation program improved the retention of ACLS guidelines better than textbook review.[11] Also, results from a systematic review concluded that multifaceted interventions for changing physicians' behaviour were effective.[6] The use of audit and feedback, education, and clinical guidelines to prevent postoperative nausea and vomiting (PONV) and postoperative pain were effective in changing anaesthetists' prescribing patterns[12,13] and improving patient outcome.[14]

Applying evidence from systematic reviews to individual patients

After critical appraisal of systematic reviews, questions of transferability of the average treatment effect and clinical applicability remain. Encouragingly, treatment found to be beneficial in a narrow range of patients can have broader application in actual practice.[15] Furthermore, differences between study participants and patients in the real-world practice tend to be quantitative (differences in degree of risk of the outcome) rather than qualitative (no risk of outcome).[15]

Transferability and applicability

To consider how transferable the results are from systematic reviews, three questions need to be addressed:[16]

- What are the beneficial and harmful effects of the intervention?
- Are there variations in the relative treatment effect?
- How does the treatment effect vary with baseline risk level?

Applicability addresses whether a particular treatment that showed an overall benefit in a study or systematic review can be expected to convey the same benefit to an individual patient.[16] Two questions to consider when addressing how applicable the results are to individual patients are:[16]

- What are the predicted absolute risk reductions for individual patients?
- Do the expected benefits outweigh the harms?

When this framework was applied to systematic reviews of ondansetron for the prevention and/or treatment of PONV,[17] the transferability issues were well described. However, the applicability questions were poorly addressed. None of the systematic reviews reported patient preferences associated with risk–benefit ratio because there was a lack of data in the primary randomised controlled trials included in the systematic reviews.[17] More effort is required in reporting the results of meta-analysis in a way that will help anaesthetists apply the results to their daily practice. If applicability issues are addressed, we believe that this will greatly help anaesthetists to individualise treatment.

Number needed to treat

One of the most common methods of applying the results to individuals is the use of number needed to treat (NNT). The NNT is the number of patients who must receive an intervention of therapy during a specific period of time to prevent one adverse outcome or produce one positive outcome.[18] The NNT is more informative than the summary relative risk (RR) and is increasingly being reported. For example, a RR of 0·63 may represent two situations in which treatment reduces the risk of mortality: a reduction of 1% to 0·67% or a reduction from 30% to 20%. However, the corresponding NNTs are 303 and 10, respectively.

It is important to realise that the pooled NNT may be misleading because NNTs are sensitive to factors that change the baseline risk, such as the outcome considered, trends in disease risk over time, and clinical setting.[19] A more appropriate NNT can be derived by applying the relative risk reductions from treatment estimated by a meta-analysis to relevant baseline risks for different types of patients (Box 13.2).[19] This assumes that the risk reduction is constant across the range of baseline risk. Similarly, a number needed to harm (NNH) can be

---

Box 13.2 Calculating number needed to treat for high-risk and low-risk groups

The relative risk of vomiting within the first 48 hours after prophylactic 4 mg intravenous ondansetron is 0·74 (95% confidence interval 0·68–0·79).[20]

In a high-risk group:

- Baseline risk of vomiting without treatment is 80% = 0·80
- Risk of vomiting on treatment is 0·80 × 0·74 = 0·59
- Risk difference is 0·80 − 0·59 = 0·21
- NNT is 1 ÷ risk difference = 1/0·21 = 4·8
- Repeat calculation using above 95% confidence intervals (CI).
- Therefore NNT is 5 (95% CI 4–6) patients to avoid one vomiting

In a low risk group:

- Baseline risk of vomiting without treatment is 20% = 0·20
- Risk of vomiting on treatment is 0·20 × 0·74 = 0·15
- Risk difference is 0·20 − 0·15 = 0·05
- NNT is 1 ÷ risk difference = 1/0·05 − 20
- Repeat calculation using above 95% confidence intervals
- Therefore NNT is 20 (95% CI 16 to 24) patients to avoid one vomiting

From[17] Reproduced with permission from Lippincott Williams & Wilkins, 2002

---

derived in the same way. The likelihood of being helped versus harmed (LHH) can be expressed as (1/NNT):(1/NNH) and adjusted according to patient's values.[21] For example, LHH of 8:1 suggests that the treatment is eight times as likely to help the patient as to harm the patient.

Which patients will benefit?

Applying a risk–benefit approach[22] is useful when deciding which patients will benefit from an intervention. This requires data from a meta-analysis, cohort study, and patient preferences. The example below is similar to the one published in our recent paper.[17]

We illustrate how this approach can be used to decide which patients will benefit most from the use of intravenous ondansetron 4 mg to prevent postoperative vomiting in the first 48 hours. The absolute relative risk reduction of postoperative vomiting associated with ondansetron was 20% (17–24%) with a mean control rate of 56% (54–59%).[20] In this example, harm is defined as the incidence of headache. Using the results from the same systematic review,[20] the excess risk of headache was 1% (−1–3%). Patient preferences and how they weight benefit and harm should be obtained whenever possible and incorporated into the decision-making process. The monetary

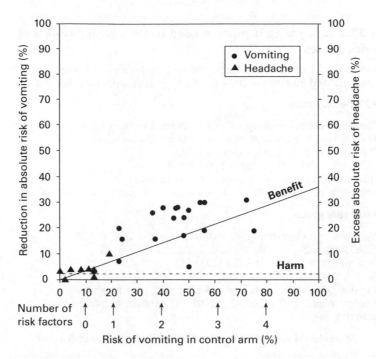

Figure 13.2 Benefit compared with harm for the prophylaxis of vomiting (0–48 hours) by an intravenous dose of ondansetron 4 mg. Data taken from[20]. The number of risk factors is described in[23]

value given to decreasing and eliminating emesis compared with experiencing headache was a 1:1 ratio.[24] When the above data are plotted (Figure 13.2), the point at which the line of benefit and the line of harm crossed was defined as the threshold. Net benefit occurred only when the line of benefit was above the threshold of 5% risk of vomiting. If, however, the patient weighted the benefit:harm ratio as 1:10, then the threshold is set at 27% risk of vomiting.

The Apfel risk score for predicting PONV is one of the most valid and reliable models.[23] The four predictors of PONV were female gender, history of motion sickness or PONV, non-smoker, and the use of postoperative opioids.[23] If none, one, two, three, or four of these risk factors were present, the incidences of PONV were 10, 21, 39, 61, and 79% respectively.[23] When these are plotted in Figure 13.2, patients at low risk (< 10%) would not benefit from ondansetron prophylaxis and may even experience more harm than benefit. If however, the patient weighted the benefit:harm ratio as 1:10, then only those with two or more risk factors would benefit from ondansetron prophylaxis.

The method outlined above is not intended to replace clinical judgment but, rather, to supplement it. In clinical practice, many other factors, including costs, need to be taken into account when making a clinical decision.

Conclusions

There is a need for improved reporting and conduct of systematic reviews in a way that will help anaesthetists to individualise treatment. In particular, applicability issues need to be discussed so that anaesthetists have a clear assessment of benefits versus harms. Often this requires multiple sources of evidence as well as obtaining patient preferences. Timely dissemination of evidence by known effective strategies is also needed if evidence is to be implemented successfully into clinical practice. Only then can evidence-based patient-centred decisions be made.

References

1. Myles PS, Bain DL, Johnson F, McMahon R. Is anaesthesia evidence-based? A survey of anaesthetic practice. *Br J Anaesth* 1999;**82**:591–5.
2. Sheldon TA, Guyatt GH, Haines A. Getting research findings into practice: when to act on the evidence. *BMJ* 1998;**317**:139–42.
3. Antman EM, Lau J, Kupelnick B, Mosteller F, Chalmers TC. A comparison of results of meta-analyses of randomized control trials and recommendations of clinical experts: treatments for myocardial infarction. *JAMA* 1992;**268**:240–8.
4. Choi PT, Halpern SH, Malik N, Jadad AR, Tramèr MR, Walder B. Examining the evidence in anesthesia literature: a critical appraisal of systematic reviews. *Anesth Analg* 2001;**92**:700–9.
5. Pedersen T, Møller AM, Cracknell J. The mission of the Cochrane Anesthesia Review Group: preparing and disseminating systematic reviews of the effect of health care in anesthesiology. *Anesth Analg* 2002;**95**:1012–8.
6. Bero LA, Grilli R, Grimshaw JM, Harvey E, Oxman AD, Thomson MA. Closing the gap between research and practice: an overview of systematic reviews of interventions to promote the implementation of research findings. The Cochrane Effective Practice and Organization of Care Review Group. *BMJ* 1998;**317**:465–8.
7. Heath KJ, Jones JG. Experiences and attitudes of consultant and nontraining grade anaesthetists to continuing medical education (CME). *Anaesthesia* 1998;**53**:461–7.
8. Haines A, Donald A. Making better use of research findings. *BMJ* 1998;**317**:72–5.
9. Haynes B, Haines A. Barriers and bridges to evidence based clinical practice. *BMJ* 1998;**317**:273–6.
10. Davis DA, Thomson MA, Oxman AD, Haynes RB. Changing physician performance: a systematic review of the effect of continuing medical education strategies. *JAMA* 1995;**274**:700–5.
11. Schwid HA, Rooke GA, Ross BK, Sivarajan M. Use of a computerized advanced cardiac life support simulator improves retention of advanced cardiac life support guidelines better than a textbook review. *Crit Care Med* 1999;**27**:821–4.
12. Cohen MM, Rose DK, Yee DA. Changing anesthesiologists' practice patterns. can it be done? *Anesthesiology* 1996;**85**:260–9.
13. Rose DK, Cohen MM, Yee DA. Changing the practice of pain management. *Anesth Analg* 1997;**84**:764–72.

14. Harmer M, Davies KA. The effect of education, assessment and a standardised prescription on postoperative pain management: the value of clinical audit in the establishment of acute pain services. *Anaesthesia* 1998;**53**:424–30.
15. McAlister FA. Applying the results of systematic reviews at the bedside. In: Egger M, Davey SG, Altman DG, eds. *Systematic reviews in health care: meta-analysis in context.* London: BMJ Publishing Group, 2001;373–85.
16. O'Connell A, Glasziou P, Hill S, Sarunac J, Lowe J, Henry D. Results of clinical trials and systematic reviews: to whom do they apply? In: Stevens A, Abrams K, Brazier J, Fitzpatrick R, Lilford R, eds. *The advanced handbook of methods in evidence based healthcare.* London: Sage Publications, 2001;56–72.
17. Lee A, Gin T. Applying the results of quantitative systematic reviews to clinical practice. *Anesth Analg* 2002;**94**:372–7.
18. Laupacis A, Sackett DL, Roberts RS. An assessment of clinically useful measures of the consequences of treatment. *N Engl J Med* 1988;**318**:1728–33.
19. Smeeth L, Haines A, Ebrahim S. Numbers needed to treat derived from meta-analyses – sometimes informative, usually misleading. *BMJ* 1999;**318**:1548–51.
20. Tramèr MR, Reynolds DJ, Moore RA, McQuay HJ. Efficacy, dose–response, and safety of ondansetron in prevention of postoperative nausea and vomiting: a quantitative systematic review of randomized placebo-controlled trials. *Anesthesiology* 1997;**87**:1277–89.
21. Guyatt G, Straus S, McAlister F, *et al.* Moving from evidence to action-incorporating patient values. In: Guyatt G, Rennie D, eds. *Users' guides to the medical literature: a manual for evidence-based clinical practice.* Chicago: American Medical Association, 2002;567–82.
22. Glasziou PP, Irwig LM. An evidence based approach to individualising treatment. *BMJ* 1995;**311**:1356–9.
23. Apfel CC, Kranke P, Eberhart LH, Roos A, Roewer N. Comparison of predictive models for postoperative nausea and vomiting. *Br J Anaesth* 2002;**88**:234–40.
24. Engoren M, Steffel C. How much will patients pay to avoid unpleasant side effects of anesthesia and surgery? *Anesthesiology* 1999;**91**:A1211.

14: Postoperative epidural analgesia and outcome – a research agenda

KATHRINE HOLTE, HENRIK KEHLET

Introduction

In recent years there has been an ongoing debate on the effects of continuous postoperative epidural analgesia on outcome. Several meta-analyses,[1-4] quantitative and qualitative reviews,[5] and large randomised trials[6-8] have been published, with conflicting results. Thus, the question *Does postoperative epidural analgesia improve postoperative outcome?* remains unanswered. In this chapter, we will discuss the advantages and pitfalls of the available meta-analyses and selected large, randomised trials, and provide recommendations for the design of future studies to clarify the effects of epidural analgesia on postoperative outcome. We will also argue that further meta-analyses and systematic reviews of previous randomised trials are not desirable, due to their suboptimal design; hence, they are unable to provide answers to relevant questions.

The superior analgesic effect of postoperative epidural analgesia including local anaesthetics is well established.[3,9] Furthermore, it is well known that single-dose epidural blockade (for *intra*-operative anaesthesia) has no stress-modifying effects in the *post*operative period.[10,11] Therefore, we only evaluate the evidence of *post*operative epidural analgesia with local anaesthetics on non-pain outcomes. Three issues are important when evaluating trials or systematic reviews aiming to investigate the effects of epidural analgesia on postoperative outcome. Firstly, the documented advantageous physiological effects of an epidural blockade are primarily based on a blockade of the afferent (from the wound) and efferent (from the central nervous system) neural pathways, thereby reducing endocrine–metabolic responses and reflexes within the autonomic nervous system.[11] In order to achieve these effects, three issues are important: the epidural blockade has to be placed at the appropriate level (that is, inputs from the wound are blocked); local anaesthetics must be applied in sufficient concentrations, as epidural opioids alone do not block afferent input or modify stress responses; and the blockade must be maintained postoperatively for an adequate period (not less than 24–48 hours, depending on the surgical insult). Without fulfilling these minimal requirements, epidural analgesia cannot be expected to have any beneficial effects. The rationale behind the potential beneficial effects of epidural analgesia on postoperative outcome is the well documented stress-reducing effects of epidural local anaesthetics when applied as indicated above.[11] Secondly, there are major differences between the physiological effects of epidural analgesia. It is most efficient in procedures carried out on the lower body because of a more sufficient blockade of the afferent input and surgical stress responses, which can be only partially blocked in upper abdominal surgery.[10,11] Thus, when evaluating trials with epidural analgesia, it is important to standardise the surgical procedure in relation to the type of epidural analgesia – that is, the level at which the analgesic is placed and its composition. Thirdly, it is imperative that the perioperative management in these studies is standardised and revised to ensure that the beneficial physiological effects of postoperative epidural analgesia are used to improve patient recovery efficiently. For example, the dynamic pain relief that is achieved must be incorporated into an enforced mobilisation programme because pain relief *per se* does not automatically improve outcome.[5] Also, the positive effects of epidural local anaesthetics on postoperative ileus[3,12] must be utilised by enforcing early oral feeding and avoiding the use of nasogastric tubes so that maximal beneficial effects can be obtained.[13]

Meta-analyses and systematic reviews

To date, the largest meta-analysis on the effects of neural blockade on postoperative outcome included 141 trials with 9559 patients randomised to spinal/epidural anaesthesia with or without additional general anaesthesia versus general anaesthesia alone.[4] The primary end points of the analysis were morbidity and mortality, and the results were largely in favour of spinal/epidural anaesthesia with a 30% reduction in mortality, a 44% reduction in deep venous thrombosis, a 55% reduction in pulmonary embolism, and a 39% reduction in pneumonia with intra-operative spinal or epidural anaesthesia compared with general anaesthetic regimens.[4] However, the majority of positive findings in this meta-analysis came from studies in procedures on the lower extremity with a single-dose epidural or spinal anaesthesia, and were thereby in accordance with the more complete conduction blockade obtained by epidural blockade in lower extremity procedures.[11] Furthermore, different surgical procedures were pooled and the composition of the drugs used for neural blockade was variable, as was the level and duration (postoperatively) of the neural block. Also, mortality was not an end point in many of the included original studies. Thus, from a methodological viewpoint, the strengths of this meta-analysis are the pooling of all available data and the analysis of postoperative outcome after spinal/epidural anaesthesia *per se*. However, the lack of specific information from a large number of studies makes the results difficult to interpret with respect to recommendations for daily practice, except for procedures involving the lower body.

Another meta-analysis compared the effect of *continuous* postoperative epidural analgesia with systemic analgesia on pulmonary function and complications.[1] Epidural opioids were found to reduce the relative risk of atelectasis (but *not* pneumonia) to 53% compared with systemic opioids (11 studies available), whereas epidural local anaesthetics reduced the relative risk of pulmonary infection to 36% (five studies available) and the relative risk of pulmonary complications overall to 58% (six studies available).[1] However, the analysis included orthopaedic, abdominal, and thoracic surgery, which may have different outcomes due to different physiological effects of thoracic and lumbar epidural analgesia.[1] These results were largely confirmed by another systematic review describing a significant reduction in pulmonary complications with *continuous* postoperative epidural local anaesthetics, or mixtures of local anaesthetics and opioids, in abdominal procedures (from 16·7 to 10·4%) and with postoperative epidural opioids only in thoracic procedures (from 31·1 to 14·6%).[5]

A meta-analysis compared continuous postoperative epidural analgesia for >24 hours with systemic opioid analgesia in a variety of surgical procedures. It showed a significant reduction in postoperative myocardial infarction (from 6·3 to 2·5%) in patients receiving epidural analgesia (11 studies with 1173 patients), with no significant difference in in-hospital death rates.[2] A subgroup analysis found that the reduction in postoperative myocardial infarction was achieved with *thoracic* epidural, as opposed to lumbar epidural, analgesia. Only studies with perioperative death and myocardial infarction as primary outcomes were included; however, data were obtained from different epidural regimens and surgical procedures (upper/lower body), which hindered the interpretation of the results.

Another systematic review of studies in abdominal surgery with epidural analgesia only (local anaesthetics or mixtures of local anaesthetics and opioids) found a non-significant reduction in cardiac complications (from 24·5 to 16·4%) with epidural analgesia.[5]

A Cochrane meta-analysis concluded that continuous epidural local anaesthetics reduced postoperative ileus compared with systemic opioid administration[3] – a finding that is supported by several other semiquantitative reviews.[12,14] Here, subgroup analyses were made according to various outcome assessments and epidural regimens. However, the heterogeneity of the assessed studies was substantial, and most studies involved a small number of patients, thus rendering clinically valid conclusions difficult. Nevertheless, epidural opioids alone do not reduce ileus.[3,12,15] So far, the limited data suggest that low doses of epidural local anaesthetic–opioid combinations do reduce ileus, although more data are required.[3,12,15,16]

In summary, these meta-analyses suggest that continuous postoperative epidural analgesia may have beneficial effects on some aspects of outcome. However, these meta-analyses were computed by summarising results from various trials that had substantial differences in design (the use of epidural opioids and epidural local anaesthetics or mixtures) and in surgical procedures, which were often analysed together as a group. When attempting subgroup analysis with an identical type of surgery and epidural dosage regimens, the amount of data available precludes a formal meta-analysis. Furthermore, the often strict requirements of methodology in such formal meta-analyses may lead to the exclusion of a substantial number of trials that would otherwise be valid (for example, trials excluded because of pseudo-randomisation), rendering the number of available studies even smaller. Thus, the heterogeneity of the available studies makes a scientifically and clinically valid meta-analysis of the effects of continuous epidural analgesia on outcome impossible. For these reasons alone it is doubtful whether new meta-analyses of these old (together with a few more recent) data will provide any substantial new information on this topic.

Large, randomised clinical trials

Most randomised clinical trials of epidural analgesia and outcome have been underpowered to show a potential and significant reduction in perioperative morbidity and/or mortality. Owing to the large variability in the existing studies, diverging results have come from meta-analyses, as discussed above. Therefore, it has been suggested that large, randomised clinical trials should be conducted. During the past two years, three large, randomised clinical trials aiming to evaluate the effects of epidural analgesia on postoperative outcome have been published.

In one trial, the effects of epidural opioids were evaluated in 1021 patients undergoing four types of major abdominal surgery (aortic, gastric, biliary, colonic).[8] No differences in death or major complications were found between the groups, except following a subgroup analysis in patients undergoing aortic surgery. In this case, epidural analgesia reduced the overall incidence of death and major complications (mainly achieved by a reduction in respiratory failure and myocardial infarction) from 37 to 22%. However, these largely negative results are not surprising, despite the better postoperative pain relief achieved with the epidural regimen, as only epidural opioids were used, which do not inhibit surgical stress responses,[11] reduce ileus,[3,15] or provide other substantial benefits compared with systemic opioids.[1] Furthermore, there was no information available on postoperative care principles.

In another randomised trial published recently, no benefits of postoperative epidural analgesia with mixtures of local anaesthetics and opioids versus opioid-based analgesia were found in 168 patients undergoing abdominal aortic surgery.[7] Although many aspects of the study design were carefully planned, the epidural may not have blocked the adequate segments, and the concentration of local anaesthetics was low, thereby merely reflecting an epidural opioid regimen. Thus, the lack of benefit of the epidural analgesia in this study – and the lack of improved pain relief with epidural analgesia compared with systemic analgesia – is hardly surprising. Although principles of care were well described in the study, they were rather conservative with the use of nasogastric tubes and the slow stepwise institution of oral feeding, thereby not taking full advantage of the well documented ileus-reducing effects of sufficient doses of epidural local anaesthetics.[12]

In a large, prospective, randomised multicentre trial in 915 high-risk patients undergoing abdominal surgery, postoperative outcomes were not reduced by epidural analgesia, except for an improvement in analgesia and a reduction in respiratory failure.[6] In this study, the administration of epidural analgesia was not standardised (no specific mention of the level of epidural blockade, dose of local anaesthetics, or dose of epidural opioids was given), thus hindering further interpretation.[6,17] Furthermore, there was a high failure rate of the epidural regimen (in 222 of 447 patients; the catheters were withdrawn prematurely, never inserted, or inserted postoperatively), and very different operations ranging from hysterectomy to oesophagectomy were included.[6] Finally, there was no information on the principles of postoperative care.[6,17]

In summary, data from the available large, randomised studies are difficult to interpret due to obvious flaws in study design. To date, no adequately powered studies applying an optimal epidural analgesia and evaluating postoperative outcome exist and where the postoperative care plans are revised to take advantage of the beneficial physiological effects of epidural analgesia.

Strategies for future studies
of epidural analgesia and postoperative outcome

From the data available from large, randomised clinical trials, meta-analyses, and systematic reviews on the effect of continuous postoperative epidural analgesia on surgical outcome, the overall effects on morbidity, hospital stay, and convalescence have been limited, except for a reduction in pulmonary morbidity and ileus.[1–3,5–8,12,15] By contrast, comparative studies in lower body procedures have suggested a positive effect on allover morbidity and mortality by the provision of intraoperative regional blocks versus general anaesthesia.[4]

A continuous epidural analgesia including local anaesthetics has been shown convincingly to have several advantageous physiological effects, including efficient dynamic pain relief,[9] improvement of protein economy,[10,11] reduction in ileus[3,12,16] as well as improvement in postoperative pulmonary function,[11] and decrease in cardiac demands.[11] It is, therefore, surprising that these effects have not translated into a more clear-cut demonstration of improved outcome in major operations. There may be two explanations for the discrepancy between the physiological data and the clinical morbidity outcome effects. It may be that continuous postoperative epidural analgesia has no beneficial effect on postoperative morbidity (except for pulmonary outcome and ileus), or the potential advantageous clinical effects have been obscured by factors in perioperative care management that do not take full advantage of the physiological effects of epidural analgesia.

As a working hypothesis, the second explanation may be more constructive and is probably correct. Thus, several recent studies have clearly shown that postoperative outcome is determined by multiple factors involved in perioperative care[13,18–20] including patient information, stress reduction, pain relief, mobilisation, and early nutrition.[21] Several of these factors are positively achieved or supported by a continuous postoperative epidural regimen, but it is noticeable that the hitherto available randomised studies have not included such a revision of the perioperative care programme towards enforced early multimodal rehabilitation.[13] Thus, it may be thought-provoking that studies with a revision of the perioperative programme have decreased hospital stay to about three days after elective aortic surgery without using epidural analgesia,[22] which is significantly less than the 7–10 days reported in the randomised studies on epidural analgesia.[5] These results clearly indicate that factors other than epidural analgesia must be controlled and included in future trials of epidural analgesia and outcome. Similar findings have been observed with fast-track pulmonary resections, with postoperative hospital stays of between one and five days,[23,24] and in elderly high-risk patients undergoing colonic surgery, where a multimodal rehabilitation programme including continuous thoracic epidural analgesia decreased hospital stay to two to three days.[18] In later studies, the advantages of a multimodal rehabilitation regimen on pulmonary function, nocturnal hypoxaemia, exercise capacity, and preservation of lean body mass were documented.[25] In a recent small-scale ($n = 64$) randomised study comparing continuous thoracic epidural analgesia with patient-controlled analgesia in patients undergoing colonic surgery,[16] advantageous effects of epidural analgesia on pain and ileus were again confirmed. In addition, reduced fatigue, increased mobilisation and exercise capacity (six-minute walking test), as well as increased quality of life (SF-36), were found three to six weeks postoperatively. It must be emphasised that this trial is so far the best randomised trial, as it included revised perioperative care principles adjusted to recent scientific data[13] with no routine use of nasogastric tubes, early oral feeding, and mobilisation to facilitate the well known positive physiological effects of epidural analgesia on outcome.[5] Finally, a fast-track multimodal rehabilitation programme including epidural analgesia decreased hospital stay after open abdominal hysterectomy to about two days,[26] which again is less than reported previously in randomised trials comparing epidural with general anaesthesia for this operation.[5]

These observations, mostly from exploratory non-randomised trials, show that postoperative outcome is determined by multiple factors. They suggest, therefore, that previous randomised trials on epidural anaesthesia and postoperative outcome have a suboptimal design as they did not include a revised perioperative care regimen that aims to enhance recovery through the beneficial physiological effects of epidural analgesia. In addition to factors such as patient information, stress reduction, optimised pain relief, and enforced mobilisation and oral nutrition,[21] several other factors have to be considered and included in future randomised trials on epidural analgesia and outcome. Thus, careful attention to the provided fluid regimen is important, as fluid excess may increase the risk of postoperative morbidity.[27] This may be particularly relevant in major abdominal procedures, as fluid excess may also prolong postoperative ileus.[28] Again, randomised clinical trials have often included the administration of large volumes of fluid[27] or not mentioned fluid administration, thereby precluding sufficient interpretation of data.

In summary, the evolving concept of fast-track surgery and multimodal postoperative rehabilitation programmes[13] with demonstrated improved outcomes and reduction of postoperative hospital stay indicates that previous efforts to show an improvement in postoperative outcome after major operations by continuous epidural analgesia may have had a faulty design, thereby precluding sufficient interpretation and assessment of the topic. Hopefully, future randomised trials will include a revised multimodal programme aiming to enhance recovery, and thereby providing a rational basis to answer whether continuous epidural postoperative analgesia will or will not improve postoperative outcome following major operations. Consequently, further analyses of clinical studies may not be meaningful, as they are unlikely to provide valid answers to the topic.

Acknowledgement

Supported by a grant from the University of Copenhagen and the Danish Research Council (No 22-01-0160).

References

1. Ballantyne JC, Carr DB, deFerranti S, *et al*. The comparative effects of postoperative analgesic therapies on pulmonary outcome: cumulative meta-analyses of randomized, controlled trials. *Anesth Analg* 1998;**86**:598–612.
2. Beattie WS, Badner NH, Choi P. Epidural analgesia reduces postoperative myocardial infarction: a meta-analysis. *Anesth Analg* 2001;**93**:853–8.
3. Jorgensen H, Wetterslev J, Møiniche S, Dahl JB. Epidural local anaesthetics versus opioid-based analgesic regimens on postoperative gastrointestinal paralysis, PONV and pain after abdominal surgery (Cochrane Review). In: Cochrane Collaboration. *Cochrane Library*. Issue 1. Oxford: Update Software, 2002.
4. Rodgers A, Walker N, Schug S, *et al*. Reduction of postoperative mortality and morbidity with epidural or spinal anaesthesia: results from overview of randomised trials. *BMJ* 2000;**321**:1493–7.
5. Kehlet H, Holte K. Effect of postoperative analgesia on surgical outcome. *Br J Anaesth* 2001;**87**:62–72.
6. Rigg JR, Jamrozik K, Myles PS, *et al*. Epidural anaesthesia and analgesia and outcome of major surgery: a randomised trial. *Lancet* 2002;**359**:1276–82.
7. Norris EJ, Beattie C, Perler BA, *et al*. Double-masked randomized trial comparing alternate combinations of intraoperative anesthesia and postoperative analgesia in abdominal aortic surgery. *Anesthesiology* 2001;**95**:1054–67.
8. Park WY, Thompson JS, Lee KK. Effect of epidural anesthesia and analgesia on perioperative outcome: a randomized, controlled Veterans Affairs cooperative study. *Ann Surg* 2001;**234**:560–9.
9. Wheatley RG, Schug SA, Watson D. Safety and efficacy of postoperative epidural analgesia. *Br J Anaesth* 2001;**87**:47–61.
10. Holte K, Kehlet H. Epidural anaesthesia and analgesia – effects on surgical stress responses and implications for postoperative nutrition. *Clin Nutr* 2002;**21**:199–206.
11. Kehlet H. Modification of responses to surgery by neural blockade: clinical implications. In: Cousins MJ, Bridenbaugh PS, eds. *Neural blockade in clinical anesthesia and management of pain, 3rd ed*. Philadelphia, Pennsylvania: Lippincott-Raven, 1998;129–75.
12. Holte K, Kehlet H. Postoperative ileus: a preventable event. *Br J Surg* 2000;**87**: 1480–93.
13. Kehlet H, Wilmore DW. Multimodal strategies to improve surgical outcome. *Am J Surg* 2002;**183**:630–41.
14. Kehlet H, Holte K. Review of postoperative ileus. *Am J Surg* 2001;**182**:3S–10S.
15. Holte K, Kehlet H. Postoperative ileus: progress towards effective management. *Drugs* 2002;**62**:2603–15.
16. Carli F, Mayo N, Klubien K, Schricker T, Trudel J, Belliveau P. Epidural analgesia enhances functional exercise capacity and health-related quality of life after colonic surgery: results of a randomized trial. *Anesthesiology* 2002;**97**:540–9.
17. Rigg JR, Jamrozik K, Myles PS, *et al*. Design of the multicenter Australian study of epidural anesthesia and analgesia in major surgery: the MASTER trial. *Control Clin Trials* 2000;**21**:244–56.
18. Basse L, Hjort JD, Billesbolle P, Werner M, Kehlet H. A clinical pathway to accelerate recovery after colonic resection. *Ann Surg* 2000;**232**:51–7.
19. Basse L, Billesbolle P, Kehlet H. Early recovery after abdominal rectopexy with multimodal rehabilitation. *Dis Colon Rectum* 2002;**45**:195–9.
20. Basse L, Jacobsen DH, Billesbolle P, Kehlet H. Colostomy closure after Hartmann's procedure with fast-track rehabilitation. *Dis Colon Rectum* 2002;**45**:1661–4.

21. Kehlet H. Multimodal approach to control postoperative pathophysiology and rehabilitation. *Br J Anaesth* 1997;**78**:606–17.
22. Podore PC, Throop EB. Infrarenal aortic surgery with a 3-day hospital stay: a report on success with a clinical pathway. *J Vasc Surg* 1999;**29**:787–92.
23. Cerfolio RJ, Pickens A, Bass C, Katholi C. Fast-tracking pulmonary resections. *J Thorac Cardiovasc Surg* 2001;**122**:318–24.
24. Tovar EA. One-day admission for major lung resections in septuagenarians and octogenarians: a comparative study with a younger cohort. *Eur J Cardiothorac Surg* 2001;**20**:449–53.
25. Basse L, Raskov HH, Hjort JD, *et al.* Accelerated postoperative recovery programme after colonic resection improves physical performance, pulmonary function and body composition. *Br J Surg* 2002;**89**:446–53.
26. Moller C, Kehlet H, Friland SG, Schouenborg LO, Lund C, Ottesen B. Fast track hysterectomy. *Eur J Obstet Gynecol Reprod Biol* 2001;**98**:18–22.
27. Holte K, Sharrock NE, Kehlet H. Pathophysiology and clinical implications of perioperative fluid excess. *Br J Anaesth* 2002;**89**:622–32.
28. Lobo DN, Bostock KA, Neal KR, Perkins AC, Rowlands BJ, Allison SP. Effect of salt and water balance on recovery of gastrointestinal function after elective colonic resection: a randomised controlled trial. *Lancet* 2002;**359**:1812–8.

Index

Note: *v* denotes differential diagnosis or comparisons
Abbreviations: PONV, postoperative nausea and vomiting; RCT, randomised controlled trial